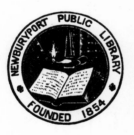

Making Babies in the '80s

RENÉE ROSE SHIELD

Making Babies in the '80s

Common Sense for New Parents

THE HARVARD COMMON PRESS

HARVARD AND BOSTON, MASSACHUSETTS

The Harvard Common Press
535 Albany Street
Boston, Massachusetts 02118

Printed in the United States of America.

Library of Congress Cataloging in Publication Data

Shield, Renée Rose.
　　Making babies in the '80s.

　　1. Parenting—Psychological aspects.　2. Pregnant
women—Psychology.　3. Infants.　4. Family—
Psychological aspects.　I. Title.　II. Title: Making
babies in the eighties.
HQ755.83.S54　1983　　　　306.8'5　　　　83–10675
ISBN O–916782–41–7

Cover design by Laurie Dolphin
Cover photo by Ben Dolphin

10　9　8　7　6　5　4　3　2　1

To Paul, my co-conspirator;
to Sonja, Aaron, and David, my raw data;
and to my parents, who told me to eat first.

Contents

Preface

This book was written following the birth of our third child. Somehow, his birth freed me to recognize a number of concerns that had been brewing in me since the birth of our first child five years earlier.

One thing I discovered by having children was that the advice I was offered all the time was not helpful and furthermore gave the mistaken message that there are certain right ways to conduct a pregnancy, have a baby, and bring up a child.

Another discovery I made was that despite the enhanced freedom and choice that women have nowadays, the alternatives available are closely bound by cultural expectations. Because these expectations are masked by an ideology of choice, decision making is confusing and constrained.

We recognize these tacit expectations when we do

not fulfill them. If you decide to bottle-feed your infant these days, for example, you will most likely be asked to explain why. If, on the contrary, you intend to breast-feed, no explanation will be necessary.

When you marry, others often ask you when you will have children. In our case, when we had our daughter, people inquired when we were going to provide her with a little brother. This happened to fit our plans, and, nicely, we soon had a son, which suited everyone. Then the questions stopped; we had fulfilled the cultural quota.

When I became pregnant with number three, people asked whether "it" was a mistake or not. And when number three was born, the usual congratulations were always followed immediately by "That's *it*, right? Your family is complete, right?" We learned from these frequent remarks that we'd transgressed slightly beyond the proper limits, and we'd better stop right there if we didn't want a lot of explaining to do. A terrific side-effect, however, of having our third child was that everyone stopped offering advice. That was worth it in itself.

To make good decisions you have to recognize the covert and sometimes overt tyrannies and stick up for what you want.

In a wonderfully happy coincidence, my sister was pregnant with her first child while I was pregnant with my third. We would talk often on the phone, avidly comparing symptoms, feelings, hopes, concerns. We were immensely reassured to discover that we shared many worries. This commonality dramatized our sister-liness, and in expressing these concerns to each other, we rendered them harmless. They became funny and manageable.

But here I was on my third child, and sharing some of my sister's worries! Shouldn't I have gotten beyond this kind of thing? Well, yes and no, I found. Cecily was reassured to know that I had worries she thought others would consider ridiculous in herself. And I found out that I *had* gotten over some anxieties and unrealistic expectations of a first pregnancy, and I shared my understandings with her. She asked me nervously during one phone call if I was practicing my breathing or not. When I laughingly told her no, she confided that she wasn't either, and we decided that we would both flunk. Finding out that we had both assumed we should be doing our homework, somehow striving for excellence in our pregnancies, suddenly made the worry about breathing exercises seem ridiculous and irrelevant.

She and I went on the layette trip together, and it was in the department store that it struck me: I had no idea what cotton balls were for and, after all my "experience," I still didn't know a kimono from a sacque. But the thing I knew that Cecily didn't yet was that it made no difference. And this I could tell her.

This book is primarily for those of you who lack the advice and support of a big sister or a good friend who's been through the process of having a baby already. I want to tell you that there's no perfect way to behave or feel. You have to find what works and do it. You need to trust yourself, and not try to control the process that's bigger than you. And that's about it.

My point of view comes, of course, from my own

experience. Though this book is mainly intended for two-parent, nonadoptive families, the philosophy expressed in these pages excludes neither the single parent nor the adoptive parent. Many of the concerns important in pregnancy are also central to parenting, and I therefore think it is important to treat the two processes together. If you are pregnant, married or not, you are getting previews of the parenting experience. And if you have just adopted your newborn, you are certainly faced with the same uproar in your home that someone who has just given birth faces. It hardly matters whether the child has your blue eyes or not.

A note on the timing of your reading. In one of the chapters that follow I mention that you may want to know things only when you want to know them. In this light I find myself wanting to warn prospective parents against reading the sections about being with the newborn at home. Maybe they will scare you? I intend the description to be reassuring; since it's an experience you can only muddle through anyway, your good intentions will get you through okay. But you be the judge of what you read when.

I have many people to thank. My brother Dan helped me especially by urging me to write these observations down in the first place. And my brother Ron was very generous many years ago by providing me with my first baby practice. This book has been read in an early draft by members of my family and numerous friends. I am grateful for the candid comments and suggestions I received, many of which I have tried to incorporate. I trust you will recognize your contributions.

Making the switch from being an independent adult to an adult caring for a dependent child may be the most shocking, the most riveting, and the most momentous transition people *choose* to make in their lives. We want to make this life change, but it is deeply challenging and threatening. It changes our image to ourselves and to others. It transforms us. It humbles us. And it is exciting. You'll see.

Introduction

This is an anti-advice advice book about having babies. Now that you are pregnant or are considering having a baby, you may be rummaging through the shelves of your bookstore or library to find the books you will need to get you through this momentous event. There are lots of these books! They tell you how to keep your figure, how to remain desirable to your husband, how to raise your child's IQ by fifty points, how to put snaps in the darts of your blouses so that you can nurse anywhere, how to breathe properly in labor, how to reject all medications in labor, how to protect your baby from the trauma of glaring lights at birth, and how, through it all, you can be the most fulfilled woman, your baby can be the most fulfilled child, and you can all live happily ever after.

This is a book about being sensible. It is addressed

to women and men of today who are intelligent, edu-
cated, serious about themselves, and knowledgeable
about their choices. Many of you are in your mid-twen-
ties or older, are working or studying for careers, and,
though you want or think you want children, you are
concerned about how to juggle parenthood with other
career options. So many of us are achievers; we want
a great many things. We have grown up with feminism,
and it has suffused us with an awareness of the overwhelming choices we have.

Feminism has been terribly important for both
women and men. Men are increasingly involved in
nurturing their children; women are increasingly exploring other career opportunities. Having children
remains a critical and vitally important thing that
women do, and it is a serious undertaking for both
parents. Being a responsible and involved mother is
more important than ever. And while men reevaluate
their own goals and careers, their roles as fathers necessarily remain crucial.

This book was written to help you wade through
some of the choices that surround you. It is hard to
choose, and it is hard to evaluate all the advice from
advice books and from other people. So the advice from
this book is to listen to yourself, respect yourself and
your husband, and decide for yourselves how to go
about having a baby and bringing up a child.

This book is addressed to men as well as women.
The husbands of pregnant women are baffled by what
their wives are going through. This book describes
some of the changes and, especially, the mix of feelings
that typically accompanies pregnancy. The book is also

for prospective and new fathers, because they share with their wives the daily decisions about the baby, and because becoming parents is difficult for them as well.

This book is not meant to be a comprehensive guide to the physiological and medical aspects of producing a child. It will not enable you to deliver your child at home, and it will not teach you how to make baby foods from wheat germ and tofu. It will not help you reduce your waistline by ten inches. It will not teach you how to educate your child at home, or how to pick the best school. It will not condemn the medical profession, nor will it pooh-pooh midwifery. It won't teach you how to make your own crib from bamboo or baby toys from nontoxic materials, or how to breathe the "right" way so you are ecstatic through labor. It *will* relieve a lot of your worries.

Paradoxically, you are at a disadvantage because you have waited, read up on, and planned this child you're going to have. You've learned too much already: since you know the body of research on neurological development, aren't you worried that if you don't stimulate the olfactory nerve of your newborn at the critical time, he'll end up with a stunted nose? The ironic thing is that knowing the literature can paralyze new parents' confidence in their own judgment.

This book assumes that you want to have a baby, that your baby will be loved, and that you will be good, conscientious parents. This book does not teach you how to love your baby more. You will know how to do that. Its purpose is to better enable you to relax about the too-perfect ideals and too-exacting standards

that you've set for yourselves. You can be highly responsible and responsive parents without being neglect-
ful of your child. Of course you want to take the best
care of your new baby that you can. This book will
help by describing concretely the things that happen
when you have a baby. The descriptions show you that
having a baby is not pure bliss or total fulfillment. By
illustrating some of the day-to-day aspects of having a
child, these descriptions should reassure you. They con-
firm that a gamut of emotions is typical—that though
you want a child, you often doubt that want. They reassure you you're normal if you are thrilled to have a
baby, but you sometimes don't want to take care of
her, and you sometimes feel awful, and you sometimes
feel as if you made a big mistake. This book attempts
to be realistic about these things because having babies
is a mixture of miracles and tedium.

This book puts the new baby in perspective. He is
a wonder of creation, and at the same time his birth is
completely mundane. Babies are born all the time. So
while you learn how to care for your baby, you should
look after yourself as well. This means that you don't
have to take all the advice books seriously. You don't
have to follow the fads of childbearing and child rearing. You can have a midwife in the hospital and take
some analgesic but no anaesthetic, or whatever seems
appropriate and safe. You can make some of your baby
foods or buy all your baby foods, depending on your
preferences. You can feed the baby on demand, or you
can hold her and let her cry for a little while. You have
lots of choices, and in most cases there are no right
answers.

Notwithstanding all the choices you have, this book makes a case for going somewhat passive in pregnancy. What this means is that the plethora of choices available today masks the fact that you do not control everything. The abundance of choices produces an ideology of control, which can actually hinder you because it sets up false expectations and assumptions about what pregnancy, delivery, and child rearing are— that they are controllable. Nonetheless, though the process is larger than you, you make important choices.

Having a baby is a wondrous thing. Having a baby is a miracle. Being a mother is a big, rewarding job. The father's role is active and involved. It's a large responsibility to have children today. Good parents are terribly important. Parents have to respect their children, and they have to respect themselves. This book tries to balance the parents with the new baby, so that in between the thrills and the pills and the spills and the frills, there is realism and integrity.

"You'll see"

It's not what you think it's going to be—that's the kicker. You've seen mothers looking harried, you've seen mothers looking blissful, you've seen mothers and fathers together with their children having fun on a picnic, going to see *Peter Pan*, arguing at Howard Johnson's, wherever, whatever. No matter what, you have formed your own opinions and you've made your own decisions about what pregnancy and child rearing are going to be like for you.

You're wrong, but so what? You can't know what it's going to be like *for you*. Women with children have told you this in various subtle and not so subtle ways. They have shielded you from hearing the details of their labors and deliveries, or they have told you everything so you'll be "prepared." They talk among themselves about pregnancy, childbirth, fathers, and children in a knowing way. When they find out you're pregnant or planning to become pregnant they congratulate you, and then they say, "You'll see."

"Are you sure you know what you're getting into?" is a favorite refrain the experienced chant to the uninitiated. Of course not! But because the experience *is* different for everyone, no one can give you advice. This is meant to be the main reassuring point of this book.

Before this decision you've made plans; then you've changed your mind and made other plans, or you've fallen into things, had good luck or bad. In most cases, if not all, you've had the idea that you were calling the shots. For instance, you decided not to go to grad school after college, but to travel in Europe and work, and then see. That's what happened, more or less. You knew how much money you had, and how much your parents were good for, and your general expectation for the time ahead was to have adventures. To that extent the unexpected was expected and, in fact, desired.

Now that you have decided to have a child, it's a different ball game. Right away people start reminding you of how much they know and how much you don't know, and a certain insidious competition manifests itself. Though you can prepare up to a point, you do not know what it is like to be a parent or to have a child until it happens. But, again, you should take this point as reassurance: since it's going to be different for you, other people's advice, dire stories, and whatnot have only limited applicability.

How-to books about pregnancy and childbirth

often miss this vital point. Another problem with many of these books is that their emphasis is almost entirely on the child. There are at least two sides to having children, and I will be talking a lot about the parents', not just the kids'. Parents are not put on this earth just to serve their children. They have rights too, even feelings. And I believe in sticking up for parents!

One reason I feel this kind of advocacy is necessary is because new mothers today are very isolated. It used to be that they were surrounded by their mothers, sisters, aunts, and so on. No longer. Now we move away from our families. Now we have friends and neighbors nearby. But it is rare that our friends live next door. We are lucky if we like our neighbors. The telephone has helped, but only so much. More and more self-help groups have arisen to fill some of the need that this isolation has caused, and they can be extremely useful. But it sure would be nice if the mothers of new mothers were around sometimes to say it's going okay, you're going to survive, and it's been done before.

How-to books about pregnancy and childbirth stress how you *can* plan, and what you *do* control. This is helpful, to an extent. There are lists, diagrams, and flow charts that tell you what to do, step by step. You start thinking the process is an orderly one, and this is not totally accurate. Although you must make choices regarding medications, diet, and other things, your decision to become pregnant means going passive to a large extent. At the same time, you have to *actively* preserve your sense of personhood and your rights all along the way—during pregnancy, in the hospital, in

dealing with your new child, and in dealing with yourself. Mothers' rights are strangely left out of most
guides. Nobody talks about passivity because it is not
youthful, and it is un-American. But I am going to talk
about these things because they are crucial.

Passivity

One of the most cherished myths of our society is that we exercise control over our individual lives. It is only when the catastrophic happens, or when the fluke occurs, that we are reminded, if only briefly, that the control is illusory. But then we recover and forget that controlling what happened was beyond our capabilities, our willpower, our endurance, our strength. This idea of control over the external environment is so strong and so ingrained that it is rarely mentioned. It is unpleasant to think that some things just happen to us. To acknowledge that they do means recognizing the limits of our resources for controlling our lives. So, for example, if I get a cold, I search back for causes to determine why. I don't just say that I was unlucky and happened to get sick. I remember the night I went barefoot in the rain, or I attribute the cold to the change of seasons, or, if I'm really desperate, I say my resistance was down. These phrases are soothing because they seem to provide reasons, though in fact they say nothing but that I *happened* to get a cold.

At odd times we are reminded of our limits and of our mortality. On birthdays we note that another year has gone by. The stunning rapidity of the year's passage, from New Year's to Thanksgiving, and the quickness with which our children grow up are ceaseless reminders of our own aging.

Sometimes we hear of the death of someone who was young, or who had everything ahead of him—in other words, a person whose death was unexpected. We take it personally. It could happen to *us*. It reminds us unceremoniously that there aren't rules, life isn't fair, life isn't under control. You live, you love, you die. Simple. We brush the unpleasant thought away quickly and get on with things.

Youth conspires with the myth of control. We think it is okay that old people die—that sick, old people die. They've lived their lives; it's their turn; it's "time." How shocking to think that old people also may feel cheated by being close to death; for them, too, it's unexpected. It's *always* unexpected.

When we are young, we believe that all is potential. We keep our options open so we can change course at will. We study a particular subject, but we know we can switch. We get attached to someone, but we keep in the back of our minds the possibility of finding someone better sometime. We get married, but we know that divorce is possible. We settle down somewhere, but only until the next move. It is unusual nowadays to decide on a career, a spouse, or a home with the idea that we'll stick it out.

For our generation, one of the hard things about turning thirty is recognizing that some choices have already been made, even if decisions have not been. That is, avoiding decisions has consequences, too. Regardless of the decisions made or not made, the thirtieth birthday arrives! Reaching the age of thirty makes it undeniable that youth will come to an end, that we must join the ranks of other people in their trek to old age. Regrettably, we are mortal too. Imagine—even though turning thirty is reprehensible, and you vowed never to do it, it happened anyway. And if you can turn thirty, you can turn forty . . .

Pregnancy, childbearing, and being a parent are, like aging or getting a cold, largely passive states. Though we plan, consider, and act to realize our ends, we don't have much control over what happens. This enterprise is humbling. You feel mortal. All the things you vowed would never happen to you might.

Passivity seems a foreign concept to women nowadays. As we explore new roles and vigorously reject old stereotypes, the idea of passivity seems reactionary and subversive. Of course, I am not advocating that women lie down and accept whatever comes their way. I do not mean that women should give up. On the contrary. Women should continue to push and achieve and strive. Yet, while women and men explore new ways of working out their lives in their jobs and at home, a lot is still beyond control. As we learn how much is possible in our lives, we feel heady and wonderful, excited and fearful. The assumption underlying the entrance of women into new jobs and roles is that we can do anything by our endurance, our willpower, our refusal to give up. Despite all the potential women have, however, we still can't control everything. We fight limitations in political and economic matters as we go about our training and our professions. But what we sometimes fail to see is that regarding our own bodies we are not in full control, either. When we are pushing ahead with our careers, our studies, and whatever, it is hard to accept that back on the home front— that is, with our bodies—just having willpower and the smarts is not enough. We have to wait, we have to wait. This seems like the old female role, the one we're rejecting, and that's why the idea is repugnant. Nonetheless, it's true. Nine whole months!

Pregnancy manuals on the market today condemn the idea of passivity. They link it with ignorance, and they banish them both. I am talking about a different kind of passivity. I am all for taking charge and being informed. This is crucial. But somehow we must understand that life is bigger than us. The control stops somewhere. When you get pregnant, you must realize that the process is taking off with or without you. You can *aid* that process by going along with it passively—that is, by not getting in its way. You control what you can, and then you let it be.

This idea can also be characterized as receptivity. It is an active acceptance, and a watchful waiting, not a state of inertia. The traditional word for pregnant women, "expectant," is most apt.

Much of this book is about the choices you have within this essentially passive state, and how you can deal with the lack of control at times. It takes practice, and it takes time.

"Deciding" to have a baby

Imagine that the two of you have completed your educations. You both have various degrees. You have negotiated how to juggle your careers; you both work and find satisfaction and frustration in what you do. You have decided that after you have gotten your careers underway you will have two children—a boy and a girl ideally. He will share the house maintenance and the child rearing, and you will either go immediately back to work after each birth or resume your career after a certain, predetermined time with the child.

It's a very nice plan. It's fair; it conforms to the cultural dogma of the day. It is decided that a spring birth will be nice because there will be no heat of the summer for an unpleasant pregnancy, and you'll be able to take the baby out right away in the warm weather. Besides, when the child enters school, you've been told, it's good if he's not too young for the class. Either an April or May birth will be fine. Okay, throw away the pills or the diaphragm, or whatever it's been. July is the target date for conception.

Now a lot of people seem to conceive the minute they stop using contraceptives. Statistics show that the younger the partners are, the more likely it is that conception will occur sooner rather than later, say within the first three months. But what you discover right away is that statistics is not where it's at. It's you.

The time for the next period approaches. Menstruation occurs. Is everything okay? You can't stop yourself from asking this question. People start to ask if you're pregnant yet (because you've told everyone your plan, after all, and they've approved it). Could something be the matter, you wonder? Is he okay, are you okay? If you've had an abortion ever, has that affected your ability to conceive? Did he experience Vietnam and Agent Orange? Do you play too many video games? Have you eaten too much bacon? Is your organic garden on some yet-to-be-discovered toxic dump? Do you have a Love Canal near you? In other words, *is something wrong*? Maybe you didn't know that it normally takes several months to conceive. Because you may have spent so much energy determining the perfect time to have a baby, you might not have understood that your control over the timing is limited. There's probably nothing wrong. You *just* have to wait.

You may have had to wait before. For a prescribed time when you'd find out whether you got the job, maybe, or for April 15, when you'd find out if you got into college or were getting a tax rebate. This time you have to wait, and you don't know for how long. It's this basic uncertainty that's hard. You may have given yourself six months to become pregnant, and you find that you've gotten pregnant right away, but that's no good because you wanted to have the baby in June—not December, just before finals. You may have had your period three times now, and so you make an appointment with the fertility expert, but you're told that you don't have anything to worry about until at least a year goes by. But you are already worried, and people are offering advice, which makes it worse. Just relax, they say helpfully. Go on a vacation and boom, it will happen. Have champagne first. You heard about Jennie who got pregnant the instant she quit her job. (But what if *you* don't get pregnant and you're stuck without a job?!) How can you not worry when already you've taken out the basal thermometer to clock ovulation, and you're busy counting the days of the cycle to know when you're most fertile, and people are calling you to find out if you need their maternity clothes yet?

The whole world seems to be full of babies—you hear of unwanted children and child abuse, and you know that thirteen-year-old girls are having children by the millions. It seems that for everyone else, it is *so* easy. And you've read that it is hard to adopt—what *if* you have to adopt? What about the fact that you're thirty-three, and maybe it's too late for everything? After all that planning to first get your education, find the right spouse, and so on. Have you missed out? If you do end up having to adopt, are there kids to adopt anymore? Will it take five years? Wait a minute, then, you'll be thirty-eight, and he'll be close to forty—yikes, you'll be old parents. Maybe you should reconsider the whole thing.

It's all rather bizarre and frightening. To top it off, people are telling you how obnoxious children are, how many problems they bring, and how they don't sleep through the night. But now all you can think of is how much you crave one of those problem makers.

It can be a confusing, unsettling, soul-searching time. Basically, after all is said, thought, and done, you have to wait. It's passive time. The best advice is to relax, but the more you try to relax, the more tense you feel. The trouble is that there is no solution because you don't have control over the process. That's what is so maddening and nerve-racking. Maybe then you try to outsmart the whole process and decide that it's really better not to have kids. They *are* a bother, and they don't sleep through the night, and later they talk back to you and turn into teenagers.

Maybe the next thing you know, you're pregnant. It's exciting. You did it. Maybe it's been one month, three months, six months, eighteen months, two years. You've fretted, or you haven't. You told people your plan, or you didn't. It's exactly the right timing or it's different from what you planned. No matter now— you're pregnant.

You start imagining the little embryo inside you. You read up on it. You figure out how many weeks you are. You schedule your first appointment with the obstetrician. Amazingly, he asks whom you've decided on for your pediatrician. (Wonderful question! You hadn't thought of that yet!) He asks if you'll breast- or bottle-feed (another wonderful, unexpected question). You're

examined, everything is all right, and you're told to return in a month.

Imagine that, you're pregnant! Everyone's excited.
You feel sick. You feel tired. Two classic symptoms of
early pregnancy. You're relieved that you have them.
You hate that you have them. You don't have the symptoms enough. You're worried that they are mild. Why
don't you feel more nauseous? Is something the matter?
Evelyn fell asleep at work every day; how come you
don't?

The simple decision to have a baby has an ironic
ramification: it means giving yourself over to passivity.
To a large extent, when and how, and if, pregnancy
happens is out of your control. There is a benefit to
recognizing and acknowledging this fact from the start.
It prepares you for the passivity inherent in the state of
pregnancy. It prepares you for the passivity necessary
for labor and delivery. And, to a considerable extent, it
gets you ready for the limited control you will exert
in bringing up one or more children.

Welcome to ambivalence

In case you haven't felt ambivalence before, you are most likely becoming quite familiar with it now. This is a normal feeling. Perhaps you may be reassured to know that ambivalence is a pregnancy symptom, too. Once you are pregnant, after all, your hormones are in an uproar. Everything is changing in your body. Preparations are being made; your body is on military alert. There is an increased blood supply; your heart is beating faster (especially when you climb stairs); your breasts feel tender. Your hip bones or rib bones may be hurting! There's lots more. It's good to read a pregnancy manual to find out about the many physiological and hormonal changes that are going on and to learn what they are about.

Ambivalence, whether caused by hormones or not, accompanies the changes your body is going through.

Your feelings of ambivalence can be startling and confusing. Now that you are pregnant, why are you wondering why you did it?

Yikes, a baby. You're not sure. Maybe you should have waited another year. After all, you and your husband don't know each other all that well. (It's been only six years that you've been together.) Things have been pretty good, but maybe they could be better. What if you had married Joe instead? Will you now have to get a babysitter just to go to the movies? How can your husband say it's just fine, and then get back to other things? How come he isn't more solicitous of you? (Why is he hovering?) Maybe the whole thing was a bad idea. Maybe you won't like being a mother at all. You're not a very patient person. Don't you have to be patient to be a good mother? Nine months is so long to wait. You wish it would happen right now—a cute, beautiful, adoring, little baby. Ooh, it will be so nice, so cozy. You'll read to her every night. You can't wait to sing lullabies. You won't be sexist. You'll teach Pilar that it's okay to be tough. She'll be on the baseball team. Jules will be allowed to cry when he's twenty-seven. He'll be taught that it's okay to be nurturing. You won't worry when he wants to wear nail polish. You'll make sure the books at school aren't sexist. Or violent. Violent books are a bad influence. No guns. No TV—it rots kids' minds. It's going to be so harmonious. Only good vibes. You'll work part time, so you'll stay fulfilled. Quality time is better than quantity time. You won't have to say no. You won't inhibit the natural curiosity and creativity of your child. You'll let him blossom and unfold naturally.

You have hopes and dreams and fears. Your husband may or may not share them. At the same time, other people are telling you their experiences, and they are offering advice and commentary. They sound so sure of themselves. And when you tell them how you think it will be for you, they smile indulgently and say, "You'll see."

It all adds up to ambivalence and confusion. It is helpful to recognize that these emotions are unavoidable. This is the reason I stress the concept of passivity. Whether you decide everything in advance or not, things change, and so do your feelings. Acknowledging ambivalence and accepting passivity prevents you from sweating it too much. Let it happen to you. You have become pregnant: your body has taken over to handle it, so don't be in your body's way. It knows how to do it. Get your doctor's advice; make the choices you need to make; try to stay healthy; and be sensible. After that, go into neutral.

Ambivalence may be uncomfortable, and it may last for quite a while. Or it could come and go. Maybe you've always made decisions comfortably and easily, and you've been counting on feeling as certain as ever. But even if you don't normally feel or haven't formerly felt much ambivalence, the fact that you do now shouldn't scare you into thinking that you have gone and done the most awful thing possible. Just blame it on hormones if you need a scapegoat, and leave it at that.

Feelings

There are all kinds of feelings in pregnancy, and a lot of them surprise you. You can be very moody, feeling elated now, and unexpectedly irritable in a few minutes. You can be feeling just fine, and your husband says something that suddenly reduces you to tears. He's totally baffled, and you're outraged.

The tears can come very easily. You feel somehow quite vulnerable. Your body sometimes seems alien, yet you're protective of it as if it's dangerous and fragile all at the same time. Your driving doesn't feel right; maybe you've become approximate about it, and that scares you because maybe you've always prided yourself on your driving precision. You're exhausted, and you can't sleep. You're excited about having a baby; you're scared to death.

It's pretty overwhelming. You just don't know

what you've gotten yourself into. How can you know? Your husband may be plenty worried too, but he hasn't been feeling the changes physiologically. (It's going to be a bigger shock to him when the baby actually comes.) You don't know what a mother is supposed to be; all you really know about that is who your own mother is, and you may be so ambivalent about her that you feel you can't use her as a resource. If you *can* talk to her, you may find her very helpful. You may feel a kinship with her for the first time in your life.

You imagine a female child, perhaps. How could your body contain a male child? A woman making a baby boy! You have a preference for one sex or the other, probably, and maybe you dream a lot. You think about yourself as a child; you remember your mother mothering you; you remember her making your siblings, perhaps. You compare yourself to her. You'll be better! You can't be as good! Your father, your husband. Your husband a father. So strange, all of it. And quite thrilling.

It's so nice to think about names and to imagine personalities that go with them. The names you're especially fond of may seem private to you. Everyone wants to know the names you're considering. You may feel that they're intruding when they want to know. The names have a magical intimacy for you.

You feel so full, so important, so productive! But are you heading for disaster? This is a no-turning-back decision that the two of you have made. What if you want to give the kid back? (Don't worry, you will at times.) What will having a baby do for your hard-won sense of personhood? Will no one take you seriously anymore? Will you take yourself seriously? Will others see only "mother" when they look at you, rather than "accountant," "writer," "therapist," "student," "lawyer," or "secretary"? How will you see yourself? Won't you be drowning in that baby? Won't you be totally taken over by the cares and pleasures of motherhood? Part of you wants to make brownies and cuddle little bodies and put bandaids on wounded knees forever. And part of you is afraid you won't escape from that, that it's a life sentence. Part of you wishes it while part of you fears it.

You've got some kind of plan, some kind of agenda, which, whether you acknowledge it or not, is going to be tested against experience. So it's an incredible gamble: you are counting on feeling certain ways and doing certain things, such as working part time or getting back to school after a few years, or incorporating the baby right into your life as it is now, full-time work and all, like that! But you *know* that you don't really know what it's going to be like. It's more than a little frightening.

This pregnancy is your and your husband's link to the future. What will your home sound like with racing kids in it? Where will the mittens get lost? Will there be enough money? Will your child feel about you as you feel about your parents?

What about your marriage? Will the baby come between you? Will you feel so caught up in the baby's needs that you become unavailable to your husband? How is he going to be with the baby? Will he really help? There will be so many things to argue about. Will you share the same ideas about discipline, and sugar, and TV, and schooling? What terrible things are you going to find out about each other? And what lovely things?

How close the two of you feel in bed, nestled like spoons, your belly against the small of his back. The two of you have created this being between you! He can feel the baby kicking at his back; he feels the pulsating rhythm of those pokes. He's shocked by the rudeness of the quick jabs. It pleases you to see his surprise and to know he feels the baby's playful movements. The two of you try to imagine that this is an elbow, this a knee skirting across your taut belly. It's funny! Push that knee back in! It pushes you at the other end of your belly now. The two of you play games with your child. Such an intimate joke you share. This is a sweet preview; one night your infant may be snuggled between you like this while you're nursing or giving the bottle.

It's a vast mix of feelings that you experience while pregnant, and they shift and change. Don't try to censor them. Acknowledge your feelings, savor them, and don't worry about them.

Pregnancy as passivity

When you find yourself newly, freshly pregnant, you face choices regarding labor and delivery, and so you become informed about the pros and cons of lots of things like medications, anaesthetics, and so on. It is important to acknowledge your own preferences, and you should consider them very seriously.

Then you settle in and wait. Each week drags by amazingly slowly. There is nothing you can do to speed things up. Yet when you think about it and read about it, the process of growing a human baby seems to go so terribly fast. The changes that a human embryo makes from week to week are staggering. It is great to read all about it, and to imagine it. But what are *you* doing in the meantime? Suffering, perhaps? Throwing up? Sleeping? Crying? All of these things? Basically, you're waiting, and letting your body do it. You should take care of yourself, even pamper yourself if you feel like it. You should respond to the signals your body is putting out, and you should try to follow what your body is doing, rather than try to lead it. If you feel very tired, lie down and take a nap. If you really don't want to eat right now, don't. If you're really hungry, eat. That kind of thing.

Your body is pregnant, and it is handling this new situation. There's so much you don't know about what is going on in there. You don't know what sex the kid is going to be. You don't know what she will look like. You don't know whether she will be healthy. You don't know whether the baby is going to be a sweet, even-tempered little darling, or whether she is going to scream her lungs out for fun every night the first month. All you know is that you are pregnant, and that you are concentrating on taking care of your pregnant body, while this *separate* organism grows on its own.

You are a vessel, I hate to say, for this separately growing organism. You do not control how the kid will turn out. That doesn't mean that you shouldn't be sensible, of course. Don't take medication unless you've cleared it with the obstetrician. Drink only a very small amount of alcohol, if any. You shouldn't smoke. It would be nice if you don't gain seventy-five pounds. It's good to exercise. Certainly, your behavior has a decided impact on this baby. But your influence is limited, nonetheless.

For example, despite your best intentions, your most favorable vibes, the best dietary habits, and so forth, you just might have a miscarriage. If it happens, it will not be your fault. It will not happen because you rode your bike, or because you're not completely sure that you want the baby, or probably even because you fell down last week. A certain percentage of all conceptions end in miscarriage. The union of the egg and the sperm isn't quite right, the conceptus is damaged in some way, the implantation on the uterine wall is not quite right, the placenta has something wrong with it, whatever. There are so many things that could go wrong. Miscarriage is so common, in fact, that it seems a wonder sometimes that babies are born at all. And, really, it is a miracle.

The chances are small that you will have a miscarriage. If you do have one, you're not unique. When someone plants a garden, a certain percentage of the seeds don't come up. Gardeners prepare for this by throwing in extra seeds. Well, human beings plant some seeds that don't come up either. It's usually neither more nor less than that.

The most common time to miscarry is in the first three months. The tenth through twelfth weeks are the prime times. If you should start to have some spotting, you call the doctor, of course. She might tell you to get to bed, or she might say you should go about whatever it is you are doing, and it might or might not happen. No matter what you do, whatever is going to happen will. But if you are spotting, this is a hard, bad time. You have to wait. If you continue to bleed, and it's bright red and clotted and you have cramps, there is a good chance that you are aborting the fetus. But, maybe not. For some reason part of the placenta breaks off sometimes, and you get some bleeding. If that's the cause, then the bleeding will stop after a few days, and everything is fine. But if your body is aborting the fetus, you might have some brown smudgy staining for a while, then nothing for a day, then a few more spots, then maybe some cramps and slightly redder staining, and so on for a few days. It's hard to wait it out to see what happens. Maybe you can have a sonogram performed; it can tell you whether the fetus is alive or not. By providing information about what's going on, this procedure can be wonderfully reassuring.

If you are going to miscarry, then it's good that it's happening. It probably means that the fetus was defective in some way, and this is nature's way of cleansing things and getting them right. If you do go through a miscarriage, of course, this awareness may be small consolation. But it just might help to know that you are not the only one: miscarriage really does happen a great deal, and it probably doesn't mean that you and your husband's ability to have a child is at all jeopardized or in question. Anyway, get yourself checked out. There probably won't be any discernible cause for the miscarriage, and most likely the obstetrician will just tell you to wait a couple of months to let your body get back to normal—and then, try again.

You can feel awful after a miscarriage. It's a very sad thing, and you might even go through a kind of mourning for the lost fetus. If you do, be assured that a great many women feel the same way. You were already getting to know that baby; you were planning and anticipating, hoping and fearing. People may be abrupt with you, and tell you how lucky you were that you miscarried. They may assail you with stories about how so-and-so didn't miscarry and had a hydrocephalic.

You hate that they do that. Can't they see that such comments are hurtful and insensitive? No, they can't. It takes a while to get over a miscarriage, so go easy on yourself, and, while you're at it, think of some good retorts to the unpleasant remarks.

Sometimes women can tell that a pregnancy is not right, and then again, lots of times everything seems just fine before a miscarriage. Some women have a sense of how their bodies are, and they may know what's coming. A lot of women know when they are pregnant, for instance, sometimes even before their periods are due. But no matter whether you sense it or you don't, you can't *control* whether you are pregnant or whether you're not, and whether you'll miscarry or whether you won't. Sure is humbling!

Maybe you're worrying a lot while you are pregnant. It's very common to do that. Partly it's hormones; partly, I suspect, it's the discomfort of having to be so passive and expectant; and partly it's realistic. After all, you can't see inside to know how the fetus looks and what's going on in there. You get checked each month, and you know that things are basically going all right. But these assurances don't tell you everything you want to know, and the plain fact is that you can't know everything you want to. If you're not worrying very much, good! If you're worrying your head off, try to take comfort in the fact that it's normal to do so. Remember that you can't do anything about the course of the pregnancy, and try to relax and forget about it.

The first three months are a very tentative time. You don't look very pregnant; the risk of miscarriage is highest; you don't feel any kicking; and normally the obstetrician can't detect any heartbeat yet. But as you get into the second trimester, things really happen. You start to look different. You need to wear maternity clothes. And when you first feel the kicking, it's incredible. Hearing the heartbeat the first time is thrilling. It is so amazing that you have a really separate, live organism in there. And it's not *you*.

Now I want to talk about the fact that it's *not* you. Imagine that. You guys had the egg and sperm, you created this thing, and it's growing in you; but little by little you get the distinct idea that it is quite separate. Separation isn't reserved for the day your baby goes off to kindergarten. It's a constant process. Your fetus may be kicking right now, and you may not want it to. You may have been used to controlling your body before you were pregnant, as when you squelched a yawn or something like that. Well, suppose this fetus is kicking up a storm, and you've stopped being entertained by it. Enough is enough, and, frankly, you'd like it to stop. But it doesn't. There's nothing you can do about it.

This is good practice. You can't stop the fetus from kicking; you can't control the kind of genetic material it's going to end up with; you can't control the kind of temperament it's going to have (even though you may be very calm, never raise your voice, and listen only to eighteenth-century chamber music); and when the kid wants to drop out of high school, you won't have much control over that, either!

You have to take care of you. Pretty soon, when the baby is born, you will be reading all those books about how to behave properly with your child and how to fulfill him perfectly. Now is the time to get into practice taking care of yourself. This isn't a joke. The fetus is a parasite. It gets everything it needs from you. You are eating for two, but the food you eat isn't always shared fairly. If you do not eat enough, or if you do not eat properly, the fetus will grab exactly what it needs anyhow. And you will be the one who isn't getting what you need. This is rather stark, but it is true. That fetus of yours already knows how to survive, and it is doing its darndest to make sure that it does. So take your cue from your potential kid and get what you need, too.

Nine months is really a long time. You watch your shape change. Sometimes you do a double take when you see yourself in the mirror. You can't believe you've gotten so big, that that's *you*. Maybe you're pleased with the way you look, and that big belly makes you feel satisfied and proud. Aren't you surprised when your belly bumps into things? Maybe at times you think you look awful, and you wish it would go away. Your shape changes much faster than your self-image does, and you notice the discrepancy when you catch yourself in the mirror. You'll probably have all kinds of feelings about yourself while you're pregnant. Maybe your husband thinks you look great, and maybe sometimes he too wishes you were back in your old shape. He has a mixture of emotions, too, you know, and in a way it's harder for him to keep up with what's happening since it is not directly, that is, *physically*, affecting him.

And what about sex? Maybe you've never felt so sexually charged. It's a relief not to have to think about birth control, and you feel so sexy being pregnant. But maybe not. Maybe you just feel like a big lummox. Or maybe you feel all revved up, but you *act* like a big lummox. You're heavy in bed. And the fetus is pressing on nerves. Or you're awfully tired. Or you have worries that sex will hurt the fetus (by the way, they're unfounded). Or the baby is kicking during sex. What nerve to interfere at times like these! It might help you and your husband if you talk about these things together— how you feel and how he feels. You can try out new positions and experiment, and you can tell the doctor about your fears and find out his views.

So sometimes you feel fine, and sometimes you don't. The heat of summer is hard; you feel much hotter than anyone else. Your legs swell; your fingers swell; you retain water; the extra weight of the baby becomes onerous. You walk funny, and your balance isn't quite right. Your back gives you trouble; you sometimes get sharp jabs of pain as the uterus stretches. You stretch your legs upon waking, and they cramp up. You sneeze and wet your pants. You have heartburn while trying to get to sleep. You might sneeze and sniffle the whole pregnancy (allergic rhinitis, it's called). You might get stretch marks. You might be itchy. Maybe you've got hemorrhoids or varicose veins, too. What a list!

You worry that all your symptoms will get worse since it's only your fifth month. Maybe this is your second child, and you feel as uncomfortable now as you did in your eighth month last time. How can you possibly get through this pregnancy, much less care for another baby? But how you feel now does not determine how you will be later. You may be pleasantly surprised. You never know. Sometimes your bothersome symptoms at five months diminish later on. And sometimes symptoms that you had in your first pregnancy never materialize in the second.

Maybe your pregnancy is very comfortable throughout, and you carry it off great. Is it your attitude? Probably not. Though your attitude and mood probably influence your symptoms and their severity, they don't determine them; there are massive physiological changes going on. And these changes may have little to do with your frame of mind, your good or bad thoughts, your behavior, or your willpower. A lot of it is just plain luck, which you don't control. So you do what you can to be more comfortable, and you get through it.

Advice—
whether you want it or not

Another thing about pregnancy and passivity is that this belly you carry around seems to be perceived as public property, and there is nothing you can do about it.

You walk into a supermarket, for example, and complete strangers feel they have the right to pat your belly. Your pregnant shape seems to give them license. Everyone talks to you. They want to know when you're due, if this is your first, and things like that. And if it *is* your first, then you're in for it.

You're a lawyer, and you're at a professional party. You tell everyone that you're two months pregnant. They're all happy for you, and all talk revolves around the pregnancy. You mention to your colleague on your left that you're nauseous, and without missing a beat he rushes in with, "Just you wait till you have a two-year-old, and you're nauseous with the second baby!" Is this helpful? Is this friendly? It's the old one-upping, put-down competition. Might be a good idea to turn to the amniocentesis conversation on your right.

People on the street will tell you definitively whether it's going to be a boy or a girl. You will learn many folk methods of determining this. It's fun to catalog them. People also voice their direst fears to you; they express their fervent hope you won't have a retarded kid, for example. Some seem compelled to tell you all the terrible stories they've ever heard about pregnant women. They relate tales of awful labors and deformed stillborns. The thing to remember is that no matter how many of these horror stories you seem to elicit from people, strangers or not, the fact that you hear them does *not* reflect on you. It doesn't mean that these things are going to happen to you. For some reason a pregnant belly seems to provoke anxiety in some people. They have to do something to alleviate the anxiety, and so they go and spill all the things they're worrying about to you. But it has to do with them, not you. Laugh about it, if you can. Get together with a pregnant friend and make a list of all the things you hear. It will help.

The pregnant woman is mysterious to others. No one knows what's inside, and everyone has to wait to find out. This creates an unease in people; they are worried that something might be wrong, but they can't see it. The mystery of the pregnant belly makes people react against what they don't know by acting sure of everything instead. So what you find is that everyone knows everything—that is, they act like they do. Everyone has an opinion, and, unfortunately, it's a vehement one. They tell you what their pediatrician did, or the neighbor lady, or the great-grandmother with the twenty-seven kids.

When people see an obviously pregnant woman, too, they know for a fact that she has had sex. Though we assume this about all the adults we know, the pregnant woman is living proof that the act has occurred. I think this blatancy bothers some, so there is tittering, and back-slapping jokes for the father, and sex-denying frilly maternity clothes with cute short sleeves and little bows for the mother.

Maybe in reaction to the sexuality you symbolize, people often treat you like the baby you're carrying. They know what's best for you. They want you to follow their advice. They want to protect you. Their treatment can be soothing, and it can be exasperating. They seem to have lost sight of who you are in all this.

People think they have the right to know your plans—the names you've picked, the sex you want, whether "it" was planned or not, whether you'll breast-feed or not. *You* can decide whether it is their prerogative to know these tidbits or not.

It dawns on you after a while that all the advice and opinions that you've collected and promised to follow are contradictory and illogical. One person tells you that it's terrible to gain over twenty pounds, but the next person tells you a horror story about some woman who gained too little weight. You hear vociferous pros and cons about sex, too—that it's bad for the baby, it brings on labor, it causes infection, or whatever.

What you have to do is sit yourself down and remind yourself that you have acquired a certain amount of education and experience, and that you are usually quite a sensible person with fairly good instincts. And you know what you do then? You decide that you are going to reject so-and-so's advice and accept the other guy's, or throw it all out as so much baloney. And you make up your own mind about some of the earth-shattering choices. Do *you* want to nurse the baby, or does everyone just expect it of you? You can check with your doctor about your questions and doubts. One thing you will discover is that the vehement pros and cons often don't matter very much. And when you understand *that*, you're home free.

This understanding will serve you in excellent stead when you actually have the baby. More on this later.

You might also have to listen to labor stories. These too masquerade as advice. Labor stories are seldom reassuring, whether their authors package them to sound that way or not. Though most labor stories are no doubt quite true, you must take them with a grain of salt. Though Joan says her labor lasted sixty hours and claims the world's record, she doesn't remember whether she started counting when her contractions became regular, or when she entered the hospital, or what. But she's adamant that it was sixty hours, nonetheless. And you're sitting there, completely unable to imagine sixty hours of anything; surely you'd never survive such an ordeal, would you? Some people do their figuring from the first twinges that eventually turned into labor, and others start from the time they get to the hospital. And so on. Try not to listen literally.

Other so-called advice is stuff like "don't raise your arms above your head, or the umbilical cord will wrap around his neck." These statements are untrue. Do what feels comfortable. It's heartening, perhaps, to recognize that, despite our belief that ours is a "civilized" culture with no superstitions, it is really full of bugaboos and superstitions, and pregnancy seems to bring them out full force in everybody. You have to wade through them and pick your way clear. Maybe you don't feel like raising your arms above your head, anyhow.

Nursing: pros and cons

Your doctor is asking you whether you will breast- or bottle-feed. You need to think about it, read up on it perhaps, talk about it with your husband certainly, and maybe also with friends. Basically, you should do what you think you will feel most comfortable with. There are advantages and disadvantages to nursing, and the same is true of bottle-feeding. So consider what you want to do, and don't be steam-rollered into anything you don't want.

Increasing numbers of women are nursing their babies nowadays, and probably for excellent reasons. You may be deluged with reports of all the advantages of nursing, and you may be surrounded by people who simply assume you won't even consider anything else. But, along with all the physical advantages (human milk is easy to digest, for example, and it contains important antibodies), there are certain disadvantages to nursing. For example, maybe *you* think the whole idea is awful, and you would be terribly uncomfortable doing it. If you really think so, you probably shouldn't do it. Or maybe your husband is adamantly against nursing. If he is, and he doesn't change his mind, that's another reason to consider not doing it.

But even if you and he think nursing is great, there are still some things that make it less than perfect. For instance, *you* are the one who has to get up at night, not him. He can't share the feeding, at least not in the very beginning when you are building up a milk supply and when, remember, you are most tired and would most welcome help in the middle of the night.

It's difficult that it's only you who feeds the baby. You may have a lot of worries as you get used to breast-feeding. Both you and the baby will have to figure it out. You can't just hand her over to someone else and say, "You feed her." You are the one who has to work out how much is enough, how much is too much, and what's right and wrong. And you have to work it out in conjunction with your baby. It takes time.

Not only is it hard on you sometimes that you are the only one feeding the baby, but it is also too bad for your husband and other members of the family that they cannot feed him at times. Feeding is a lovely thing to share, but when you are nursing, especially in the beginning, you really can't.

You also need support to breast-feed. You need to be surrounded by people who think you are doing the right thing and who keep telling you just that. Your husband and the others need to tell you that you're doing beautifully, and that everything will get easier. They should not doubt your ability to produce enough milk; they should not suggest things that may go wrong. If you don't have people around you giving this kind of support, then you may have a difficult time. If your family makes it hard on you, you'll have to kick them out, or consider bottle-feeding so they can take over more.

I think that's why so few of our mothers nursed us. Many tried and said they didn't have enough milk. They were not supported. Doctors were proclaiming the scientific advantages of formula. Breast-feeding seemed barbaric, old-fashioned, primitive. People told our mothers that their breasts would sag; they'd look all worn out and awful. So, you can imagine, when they tried to nurse us and we started to cry, if someone near them said they were doing it wrong, their milk was bad, their milk was insufficient, or whatever, it must have been pretty hard to withstand the disapproval and continue to breast-feed. It's a wonder any women breast-fed their babies in that climate. It's much easier today because there's more social approval of nursing.

If you decide to nurse, it's helpful to do a little preparation beforehand. Your doctor can probably give you some cream to massage your nipples with so they will be ready for the baby. A baby sucks hard, and your nipples feel it! In the hospital, too, they will help you (if you ask persistently), and they can give you lanolin to keep the nipples moisturized.

So you have to take care of yourself in order to nurse. This can be a bother. You leak in the beginning, and you have to wear nursing pads. Remembering to put lanolin on your nipples is another petty job to do; it's easy to forget, and your nipples hurt at times.

Nursing the baby keeps you public. You think about sex, and presto, your blouse is wet because you leaked. You go to a restaurant, and when the baby cries, you nurse him, but you find people think you're making a political statement. Some think it's wonderful that you're so "up front"; others think you should hide yourself in the bathroom. Nursing the baby in public is not a neutral act, though bottle-feeding is.

There are a lot of intangibles to nursing. You don't know how much milk the baby is getting. You don't know whether you need to nurse more frequently so you produce more. You have to try it different ways. If the doctor says you shouldn't nurse too frequently because it takes a few hours for the baby to digest the milk, then you try to do that; but if the baby is always crying, and you think she's hungry, you have to try nursing more frequently. There are no firm and fast rules. It's a learning process to get the right balance, and to get to a point where nursing is comfortable for both you and the baby.

While you nurse, you are tied down by the baby, especially in the beginning. You can't wear a lot of your clothes. You're restricted to shirts, sweaters, and dresses that button down the front. Also, sexual gratification from nursing varies a lot among women. It may not be very sexual at all for you. Or it may be, and you may be disturbed by that! You may have a whole bunch of emotions.

Also, babies get teeth. When they're teething, they're uncomfortable, and they bite. But let me tell you, this discomfort of theirs is much more uncomfortable for you!

You will still have to be prudent about what you eat and drink since everything gets in the milk. You should still check with your physician before taking medications. You shouldn't drink much alcohol. You should drink a lot of fluids, you should eat properly, and you should remember to keep taking your pregnancy vitamins. Sometimes it's a drag that everything you do still affects your baby so directly, and sometimes you wish that you and she were completely, finally, separate. But while you are breast-feeding, you and she are still physically linked.

This physical link is also the wonderful thing about nursing. *You* are the one who continues to be responsible for the growth of the infant. You're making the baby grow just as when he was in utero. In this respect nursing can be a very nice transition for you.

After nine months with a baby inside you, when all of a sudden he's outside you, the suddenness of the change (accompanied by the tremendous switch in hormones) can produce or exacerbate the blues. After the birth people hardly notice you at all, so preoccupied are they with the baby! But if you are nursing, your continuing direct physical tie with him makes you feel important. And feeling important helps decrease the blues. Maybe hormonal effects of the nursing help lessen your blue feelings, too, who knows? And nursing feels very good. It produces a fine closeness between you and your baby, and a deep sensuousness. You may feel great satisfaction, pride, and a sense of fulfillment when you nurse your baby.

The advantages of not having to do all the busy-work of bottle-feeding, like warming up formula, sterilizing bottles, carrying a lot of equipment wherever you go, and so on, are considerable as well. The simplicity of breast-feeding can be fabulous, especially at 3:00 AM. And maybe your husband will like getting the baby for you to nurse at night. This can be a lovely arrangement.

There are public expectations about whether you will nurse or not, but it's a private decision for you and your husband to make. You'll decide the right way.

Some of the other decisions

Other decisions that you will be making have to do with how to have the baby. Do you want "natural" childbirth? What about all the different analgesics and anaesthetics? It is all a long time away, but some thought has to be given to these matters, or else they will be decided for you. Give yourself time to read up on them, to talk about them. Discuss them with your doctor. Get second or third opinions if you're dissatisfied. You have a right to know all kinds of things. If the doctor is reluctant to talk about these matters, you should not be afraid to ask why. A real problem for doctors these days is that when they are asked for information, they are under pressure to divulge fully; however, untrained people are often not in a position to understand the ramifications of the bare information they receive.

A big reason one goes to a physician, after all, is to receive that physician's *interpretation* of the medical facts. When you ask him to give you the facts, or to spell out alternatives and options, he may respond with a barrage of information. The information itself is neutral; the physician's training and clinical experience provide him with reasons for a particular interpretation. Ask him to distinguish facts from interpretation for you. If you are not a physician, you do not have the same ability to make interpretations. Of course, you are becoming informed continually, and you've collected pregnancy, labor, and delivery stories. But, when you ask the physician to lay it all out for you, you may be surprised that the facts are frightening. Everything carries risk, for example. It is not all that safe to be pregnant in the first place. So when you ask for all the information, be prepared to get it. Then ask for the doctor's opinion. Together, you should agree on a course of action, how the labor and delivery should be conducted—all things going normally, of course. You should ask how he will behave should things go wrong, too.

Another thing you should try to distinguish, if you can, is the doctor's personality or bedside manner from her medical competence. A wonderfully warm physician can give bad care, and conversely, a cold fish may have superlative medical abilities. While you are an obstetrical patient, make sure the doctors treat you right, get the answers and opinions you need from them, and keep your priorities in mind.

If you are nearing the magic age of thirty-five, you are probably considering whether to have amniocentesis performed. It is generally advised that you have the procedure done if you are thirty-five or older, and many couples want it if they are approaching that age. This decision should be reached with your doctor, taking into account the risks of the procedure, your family history, whether there is genetic reason to do it, and so on. If you decide to go ahead with it, the information that results will include the sex of your baby! Now you have to decide whether and how to tell people. Do you tell just your parents? Or no one? Do you tell them that you know, but you're not divulging? Or if you do tell people the sex, doesn't it sound like the announcement of the actual birth? Won't the birth be an anticlimax? Certainly, amniocentesis and the kind of knowledge it brings is way ahead of the etiquette that people have been able to build around it. You have to make your own judgments about this as about everything else.

Have you been considering home birth? This can be a difficult decision, particularly if you hate hospitals and have your heart set on having your baby at home. It is lovely to be at home in bed, surrounded with warm, supportive people who urge you on and tell you you're doing great, but can they step-to if, heaven forbid, there is an emergency? It would be fabulous if having a baby could be cozy and romantic, but actually, it isn't those things anywhere. What's important is to end up with an intact body and a healthy baby.

Some incredibly high percentage of deliveries in the United States are totally without complication. The percentage is so high that we have come to believe that having a baby is totally safe. But the statistics, however encouraging, do not assure *you* of a completely uncomplicated birth. And this is the reason people go to a hospital to have a baby. Chances are that everything will go fine, but if something goes wrong, it goes wrong *fast*. Obstetrics is notorious for having emergencies arise lightning-fast. There may be no warning that something is wrong until it all of a sudden happens.

If you are at home and it is nearing the time for delivery, and all of a sudden someone listens to the baby's heartbeat and finds the pulse is seventy per minute instead of a normal 120 or so, it's bad news. Your baby may be strangling himself with the umbilical cord. If you are in the hospital, the people caring for you can handle this emergency (which may exhibit no warning signs beforehand). They can do a cesarean or a mid-forceps vaginal delivery, depending on your particular case. If you are at home, and you decide that you'd better use the elaborate backup system you planned and get right to the hospital, it may be too late. Your child isn't getting enough oxygen, and with any delay he could end up brain-damaged or dead.

Having a baby is a matter of life and death. You are having a baby; a *baby* is coming into the world, and it's not always as simple as it may seem. The foregoing is just an example of something that can happen at the last minute. Ask any obstetrician to give you other instances. Even if your pregnancy has been so normal that it's boring, it can *still* happen.

If you want a home birth, you should take a course to learn what the risks are and what procedures will be taken to minimize them. In such a course the preparations and dangers accompanying home births are usually very well spelled out. You might decide that the risks are too great or the numerous safeguards too burdensome.

A possible alternative is offered by the increasingly numerous birthing centers in the country. Usually located next to or across the street from a hospital, they may provide a safe setting for you if you want to avoid the hospital experience.

Certainly, a hospital isn't great. It's not like home. It's noisy. There are bright lights. The air conditioning isn't right. The loudspeakers blare. The nurses, residents, interns, and nursing and medical students are alternately friendly, abrupt, caring, insensitive, unavailable when you need them, and intrusive. This is not to say that physicians haven't also mistreated and shown insensitivity to patients. There is a lot of patronizing, and there used to be a lot more. It should just be understood that the good karma of home is not by itself enough to guarantee you a healthy newborn.

What about midwives? It's good to have more midwives in our society, especially since they now undergo training in modern medical techniques. Though midwives can be wonderfully supportive through labor and can provide much needed continuity of care, I think there's a danger in romanticizing the past when midwives did everything. Many mothers and babies were lost in the old days, and we're lucky to have our children at a time when the dangers attending childbirth can be very low. Maybe you'll opt to have a baby in the hospital with a midwife attending you, and a doctor available for backup. If this suits your inclinations, you can have the best of all worlds.

Now about "natural" childbirth. The problem with

the word natural is it's a slogan, and it stands for a slew of things. Each person means something different by it. One person means that you have no anaesthetic, no pain killers, no nothing; another means you're awake and aware enough that you witness the birth of your baby; and yet another means that your husband accompanies you in labor and delivery. It seems when you are pregnant, everyone in the whole world wants to know if you are going to have natural childbirth or not. Say yes, regardless. Then you'll be in everyone's good graces, and you can decide by yourself how you'll do it.

A lot of people mean 'Lamaze' when they talk about natural childbirth. The Lamaze method and others like it teach you breathing and relaxation exercises that greatly aid in labor and delivery. In these lessons, which husbands usually attend with their wives, the prospective parents are taught what to expect. They are instructed about what is going on in the pregnant body, and they are "prepared" for what will happen in labor and delivery. This preparation reduces fear and anxiety about the process. The husband learns how to coach. The breathing exercises help regulate the labor. The breathing exercises make the contractions more predictable and controllable; when you are concentrating on steady breathing rather than on the contractions themselves, they are less difficult to manage than they would be if you were just bracing yourself for the next one. When you aren't fighting the process you relax, and you therefore feel less pain. Also, you and your husband meet other couples in the classes, and a special camaraderie usually results. The other couples are interested in the outcome of your pregnancy and vice versa, and that's nice. Having these friends after the babies are born can be a real boost, too.

Sometimes, however, Lamaze classes give you more information than you'd like. Some women really don't want to hear all about how to take care of their episiotomies *before* they have the babies. Sometimes you are more frightened when you know everything. Many of us (most of us?) are *not* reassured by films graphically depicting what happens in labor and delivery. You may want to know things just when you want to know them, and it may not be reassuring to have too much thrown at you unsolicited. Everyone varies about this. The idea that lots of preparation and scads of information are always good is just not necessarily true.

It used to be, in the days when our mothers had us, that pregnant women had very little instruction about childbirth. In some ways this was good, because they had less to fear. (Of course, some women were petrified at not being given any information.) The obstetrician reassuringly (and perhaps condescendingly) patted the woman on her head and told her not to worry; everything would be fine. Today, we react against this kind of blanket reassurance. And in its stead we have an ideal of total disclosure and complete preparation based on the idea that full control is possible. In a way this extreme is also unreasonable—we've gone from no information to total information. Though the prevailing opinion has changed, women still have individual and idiosyncratic needs and wishes regarding exactly how much and what kind of information they want.

And men, too! Though the cultural climate of the day insists that men be present during labor and delivery, your husband may have negative feelings about it. Most men, nowadays, seem to want to be present at the birth and to support their wives through labor, but if your husband feels differently, his feelings should, after all, be considered. It just wouldn't be fair otherwise.

Increasingly, there seems to be great antipathy toward the treatment of pregnancy and delivery as a medical problem. When our mothers had us, it was assumed that the doctors knew everything and shouldn't be questioned. Now we have a massive distrust of hospitals and things medical. Now the prevalent idea is that *all* medications are bad, and that all obstetrical interventions are unnecessary. It's just not true. It would be good if we could stop vacillating between the extremes and arrive at some sensible, moderate point of view instead.

An assumption often underlying the Lamaze-type classes is that you can control what goes on. If you learn the breathing exercises, if you practice every day before labor like a good girl and boy, and if, when labor comes, you just execute what you've learned, you'll do a good job and get an "A." Of course, this is inaccurate and naive. You're *not* in school. You don't get grades. Everyone has a different threshold of pain. Yours may not be so high. Also, everyone's labor is different. Yours may be easy and fast, or it may last a long time. And there may or may not be complications. Why, you may even decide that you want some kind of painkiller! You may find that labor feels awful, *even though* you are faithfully following the exercises. A common message of these classes is that if you didn't have an esthetic experience in your labor, it was no good. Or if you "broke down" and had some Demerol, then you're a chicken. Or if you had an anaesthetic, then you don't really know what having a baby is all about. Or, heaven help us, if you should have committed that most heinous of sins and had a cesarean birth, well, then, you're a real failure, and just hope and pray that you can redeem yourself with the next birth. (In some cases vaginal deliveries are possible with subsequent births, though this is controversial.)

Though many instructors give a realistic picture of labor and delivery, these examples represent a prevalent attitude these days. We read testimonials by mothers and fathers having their second child the "natural" way, who conclude that they missed everything meaningful the first time. It is a feeling that tends to be exaggerated. After all, when he's thirteen and pimply and obnoxious, you probably won't be thinking that dimming the lights at the moment of birth had much to do with anything.

The point is, you want to have a baby, right? Just have the baby. The breathing exercises help because they regularize your thinking and divert your attention, and they help you to relax so your tension doesn't impede the process. But you may have another system that could work just as well, like counting slowly, for example. One particular breathing method is not *holy*, after all. And if you do have an analgesic or an anaesthetic, or if you end up having a cesarean, you haven't *failed*, for heaven's sake.

By the way, a lot of women who are having their first babies and who refuse any medication through the process are so exhausted by the time of delivery (because first labors are typically quite long), that they fall fast asleep at the moment of birth. So much for meaningful experiences!

It's good to read up on pregnancy, labor, and delivery, and to know what's going on. Classes that the hospital sponsors can be very good. They may be extremely large, but there's a lot of good information and opportunities to get answers to the stupid questions everyone wants someone to ask. And there's usually a tour of the hospital, so you can better imagine what your stay there will be like. The most important thing is that they show you what door to use when you get to the hospital at 2:00 AM, and they tell you other important things—to bring your insurance card, for example, and to leave your jewelry at home.

There are other choices to make. Some you can make in advance, and some you can't, such as what you'll do if there's an emergency, or if another woman is delivering in the one available birthing suite. Find out, too, about some of the other things: Do you have a choice, for example, about whether you will be given an enema? Are there pros and cons? Find out if you have to be shaved; your doctor might insist, or maybe she will consider a "mini-prep," that is, a partial shaving, perfectly sufficient.

Another decision to be made is whether or not you'll have an episiotomy. It's too bad this issue has become political. Our grandmothers had lots of damage to their urinary tracts because their tissues tore when they delivered their babies. The episiotomy is simply a cut the doctor makes to enlarge the vaginal opening slightly so that the baby's head can be born without tearing the perineum. Because a tear is ragged, it is harder to heal than a cut, more susceptible to infection, and so forth. Though the stitches of an episiotomy are notoriously itchy and uncomfortable, the clean cut is probably preferable to a possible tear. Massaging the perineum in the months before labor will make the tissues stretch more easily, reducing the chance of a tear. But the chance of tearing is still present, and it happens to some women.

Episiotomies are not a male conspiracy to control women by performing unnecessary operations on them. Some women say an episiotomy is done just so the doctor can sew you up "nice and tight for your husband" afterward. Anyone who says this should be told off, of course, and if that person is your doctor, maybe you should find a new one. But, nonetheless, an episiotomy is only an episiotomy.

If you can find a doctor (or midwife) who is willing, a possible alternative is to have the tissues massaged prior to the delivery, with the proviso that, as the baby is descending the birth canal (and according to the doctor's last-minute judgment), the episiotomy will be performed only if it looks as if there is going to be a tear. Then you avoid an unnecessary episiotomy, but you get one if it looks like you need it. This takes extra time on the part of the doctor (which is a reason he might not want to do it).

With subsequent deliveries the necessity of an episiotomy is lessened, so if you got one the first time and don't want one now, it may be possible to forego it.

Then there's the matter of anaesthesia during labor.

There are anaesthetics to knock you out so you can wake up and be told that you had a baby, but you don't remember a thing. Then there's stuff to numb you from the waist down. An epidural anaesthetic requires an anaesthesiologist monitoring you all the time, and it takes some skill to administer, so it's not done in all hospitals. Its advantages are that it can be given fairly early without stopping labor, and, though it numbs you from the waist down, it leaves you fully aware of everything. Its considerable disadvantage is that it sometimes doesn't work. A spinal anaesthetic also will numb you from the waist down, but it can be given only at the time of delivery since it will stop labor if given sooner. It can also produce the side effect of a very nasty headache if you're unlucky. You're not supposed to raise your head for twelve hours or more after it's given so that you won't get the headache. But what often happens is that, despite the nurses' instructions, they move you all around, up and down, while they give it to you, and so you get one because of them. But maybe you're really tired out from the labor, and it's time to have the baby, and you'd like just to watch the birth as if you were a spectator. So maybe get the spinal, hope you don't get the headache, put on your glasses, get the mirrors adjusted, hold your husband's hand and watch the show. It's a pretty nice reward. All of sudden, imagine, you don't feel anything, and you watch this baby being born.

Part of your preparation before labor is learning about these and other procedures and medications involved in labor and delivery. More is known every day about the possible ill effects that various medications have on the baby. You should inform yourself about these and discuss this subject with your doctor. Then you will be in a better position to make choices when you go through it.

By the way, how come no one glorifies the enduring of other painful procedures, such as having teeth worked on without anaesthesia? It is curious that going through labor and delivery with no analgesic has become such an ideal.

Something to remember is that these decisions can usually be modified or changed when you are actually in labor, when the doctors and nurses will ask you again what you want to do. So don't worry that the decisions you make now are irrevocable.

Preparing the layette

Has anyone ever told you what a layette is? No one ever told me! *Layette* is one of those words whose meaning no one is quite sure of, but preparing the layette is something everyone does before a baby is born. That's just the way it is. It basically means getting things ready before you end up with a baby. The word conjures up a picture of a lacy nursery with frilly crib sheets and lots of stuffed animals and ribbons softly fluttering around the bassinet.

What is all this stuff? You are supposed to go out and get a room fixed up this way because otherwise you won't be starting the baby out right, right?

The magazines you've been reading in the waiting room of the doctor's office contain the lists of things that you must buy so you'll be all ready. These are very interesting lists. Here is a sample:

crib mattress
fitted crib sheets (at
   least 2)
quilted pad
bumper
blanket sleeper
shoes and booties
2 or 3 crib blankets
waterproof pads
quilt
laundry hamper
rectal and room
   thermometers
nursery lamp
crib mobile and toys
scale
bassinet
bathinette
changing table
diaper bag
stroller, portable stroller,
   carriage
backpack baby carrier
front-pack baby carrier

portable crib
auto safety seat
safety gates and latches
electrical outlet covers
play pen
high chair
infant gowns (at least 2)
infant sacques (at least 2)
undershirts
bunting
kimonos
flannelized rubber pads
cloth diapers
receiving blankets
towels and washcloths
bibs
cotton balls
lotions and oils
petroleum jelly, diaper rash
   ointment, etc.
bottles, sterilizing equipment, etc.
infant seat
etc. ad infinitum

Help!

There are lots of things on layette lists that you and I have never heard of. Lots of them are unnecessary, too. First of all, don't buy much clothing because that's the kind of thing people give you as presents. Next, never get anything smaller than a six-month size; babies outgrow things quickly. Now, what is the difference between nightgowns, sacques, and kimonos? Maybe someone can tell you—I don't know. It doesn't matter too much. The principle is to get some uncomplicated lightweight things that you think a newborn might not be too uncomfortable in. Babies are little and very squirmy, and you have to change them a lot. So you don't want to have too much to fuss with, like snaps that are hard to figure out. (Baby clothes are full of ingeniously difficult snaps.)

In the foregoing incredible list are many items that duplicate one another unnecessarily. You don't need a carriage, a stroller, *and* a portable stroller. The carriage is only for tiny babies. Maybe you will decide that a portable stroller will fit all your needs, especially if it's winter and you won't be taking walks for a while. A stroller isn't as romantic as a frilly carriage, but it'll work okay. You don't need crib blankets *and* quilts *and* comforters. After they are several days old, full-term babies can handle the cold just as we do. And that's a good reason why you don't need a room thermometer. Babies don't need shoes, either. They can't walk. And when they do walk, having soft shoes or going barefoot is best. You don't *need* a scale or a nursery lamp or a crib mobile, but you could, of course, get any or all of these things if you want to.

Also, you don't need a portable crib and a bassinet (which is a small cradle for a newborn) and a dozen other variations of small-sized sleeping containers for the newborn. If you think you won't be going on too many overnights with the baby during the first few months, you may need only the portable crib, which is larger and sturdier. You can use it whenever you travel until the baby sleeps in a bed. You have to decide.

Cotton balls are on everyone's layette list. I'm not

sure why. For changing the baby, commercial wipes or a washcloth and water seem best to me. Otherwise, it's probably better for the baby if you leave all his orifices except mouth and anus alone. That is, you really don't have to clean nostrils and ears, wipe eyes, and things like that. If you do it wrong, for one thing, you can cause infection. Also, the baby hates that you do it, and you do, too.

When you go to buy things for the baby's room, you find a zillion, and it's hard to know how to choose. It's good to take someone along with you for support and camaraderie. How do you choose among the various kinds of crib mattresses, or the different kinds of crib bumpers? Basically, the mattresses are either horsehair and coils, or they are foam. If you and your husband are the allergic types, chances are your kids will be too, so it might be better to go with the foam. A salesperson will most likely be hovering around you, and he or she will tell you that a certain mattress won't last nearly as long as another. Exactly how long do you think it needs to last? You probably don't need it to last for six years of six babies, now, do you? Probably the cheapest of mattresses will last you long enough, so that a lot of these fine considerations won't matter much. Same thing with crib bumpers. With these the baby doesn't stick his arms and legs out of the crib and have trouble getting them back in again. The thickness of the bumper probably doesn't matter, but it is this kind of thing that determines the price. Maybe you just want to pick out the prettiest. That's a good way to decide.

Another thing is a bathinette. It's a separate piece

of furniture for bathing the baby. You do need a place to bathe the baby, but a sink is handy. You need a place to change and dress the baby, too, but you don't necessarily need a changing table, which is another extra piece of furniture. You need to have diapers and wipey things and a change of clothes conveniently nearby. It's good to try to picture where you will be feeding the baby, where you'll most often be changing him, and where all the stuff should go. My solution has been to get a chest of drawers for all the clothes. I put a thin narrow cushion on top of it, cover the cushion with a receiving blanket, and change the baby on that. And I put the diapers and diaper rash things on shelves above the dresser or right next to it so I can reach it all easily. This way I don't need to buy a changing table, which is flimsy and can't be used for other purposes later. My main consideration in getting the chest of drawers is the number of drawers it has and its height. The height determines how comfortable I'll be while changing the baby. You figure out your own system.

What are receiving blankets? These little things are quite useful. They are soft, small blankets, usually made of cotton or flannel. They are good to cover things with, like the changing table or the car seat, so their surfaces feel nice for the baby. In the beginning they are good to wrap the baby in so she's snug.

The flannelized rubber pads go on your lap so when you are feeding the baby, he starts to have a bowel movement, and it comes out of the diapers, it ends up on the lap pad instead of your lap. Very handy. But if you are going to be using elasticized disposable diapers (with elastic around the leg so they don't leak so readily), you might not need a lot of pads. If you are breast-feeding, the bowel movements are very loose and often come squirting out, so you've got to be prepared one way or the other.

The cloth diapers are good to have around for your shoulders. Babies spit up a lot, and it's helpful to have a diaper on your shoulder so the baby doesn't spit up on your shirt.

You should follow your pediatrician's advice when choosing among the various kinds of lotions, creams, ointments, shampoos, soaps, and so on. Maybe he'll recommend your getting something for diaper rash and that's all. Some doctors advise against lotions, creams, powders, and soaps because they can be irritating and drying. So try to withstand sophisticated and persuasive advertising regarding these items. Use your head— decide which things suit you and your style; consult the doctor and perhaps a friend whose judgment you trust.

When do you go to the store to buy all these things? You may feel reluctant to do it too soon. There are restrictions in some religions about getting anything before the baby is born, because planning for the new baby seems so presumptuous, so arrogant. You may feel this way yourself, and, while respecting these feelings, you may have to push yourself to go. It's difficult making some of the decisions. If you manage to get a few of the basics, though, you may feel better about getting the rest.

Some important things are missing from most layette lists. How about considering a rocking chair for comfort during the feedings? If you're nursing, you may want a breast pump. Also, if you are intending to breast-feed, buy nursing pads and nursing bras. You'll leak milk a lot in the beginning, and the pads will insure that the milk doesn't get through to your clothing. A swinging cradle may soothe the baby during her crying jags. And how about ear plugs for you?

When the baby gets a little bigger and starts crawling around, she puts everything in her mouth. You have to have ipecac on hand to make her throw up. Another good thing for the first year are liquid aspirin solutions, teething rings, and teething biscuits for the pain a baby feels when teething and for the fever she sometimes gets from inoculations. For the slightly older child, bandaids are the best solution to scraped knees and other real as well as imagined hurts. A night light is nice to have for both the earliest months, when the baby wakes up at night, and for later when the child may fear the dark. A vaporizer or humidifier may be advisable if your baby gets congested often. Wait and see.

Some things on the list I haven't mentioned. Layette lists like the foregoing often combine items needed for the first week with others you won't need for four months, eight months, two years. So you have to set your priorities. Some of the things obviously duplicate others; you might want to get them anyhow, or you might not. You should take any list like this with a grain of salt; it is presented as if everything on it is imperative for the new baby. A lot of it is nonsense. You'll figure it out.

You should get a few things for yourself as well.

Like perfume, scotch, and bubble bath! You'll very much appreciate your being good to yourself afterwards. You should perhaps treat yourself to some clothes that you'll be able to wear after the baby is born. I mean things that are quite a lot larger than your "normal" size. It can be very discouraging to have nothing to wear afterwards. You may feel defeated that you can wear only maternity clothes, so it might be nice to have one new, large thing to look forward to. A good friend who has been through all this can help you greatly.

Waiting for labor

Pregnancy lasts about nine months, but guess what? No one knows just exactly what it is that triggers labor. You go for your appointments in the last month, and the doctor says that you have some of the signs, all of the signs, or none of the signs. She says you're getting "effaced," you're starting to "dilate," you're not doing any of these things, or whatever, and she tells you to come back next week. Well, regardless of all that, you could go into labor today with no signs, or you could walk around for another couple of weeks with all the signs. Nobody knows what does it. I feel reassured just understanding this, but sometimes you may wish you could just *know*. You have to wait until it happens.

People call you up a lot the last month. As you get into your last two weeks before the due date, everyone is impatient. When you're "late," they can't believe it.

With every phone call that you answer, someone exclaims incredulously, "You're still *here*?" You start getting the impression that people are mad at you because you haven't "done it" yet.

Labor can begin anytime. The contractions can come while you are eating, talking, walking, sitting, or lying down, anytime, anyplace. You don't have to be asleep for your body to go into labor. Your being awake doesn't prevent your going into labor. *You* don't have anything to do with it; that is, your readiness, your willingness, your resistance, your willpower, your trepidation—none of these has anything to do with going into labor. Baking chocolate chip cookies doesn't do it, either (though it's an awfully good excuse to bake the cookies). There may be some correlation with the moon cycles, but then again, there may not be. So, you wait.

The nine months time is an average, too, you have to remember. Any time from two or three weeks before your due date till two or three weeks after your due date is normal for you to go into labor. So, you do whatever you can—bake the cookies, prepare the baby's room, pack your bag, get phone numbers ready so you can call relatives from the hospital. And continue going about your routine, because it can be quite disheartening to wait around for a baby who doesn't seem to want to be born. Maybe you think that you are the only pregnant woman in the world who it isn't going to happen to. You feel, perhaps, that just as it has taken a long time to grow into this shape, little by little it will start going away, and then medical research teams will write you up in the *New England Journal of Medicine*, and you will get on the cover of *Time*.

It helps to go about your business, to keep accepting dinner invitations and rides on bumpy roads. If you are called away into labor, great.

During your last trimester of pregnancy, you will probably wonder and worry about what labor is going to be like, and how you will know when you're in it. You've probably been having Braxton-Hicks contractions for a while now. If you've had other kids, you've been having the Braxton-Hicks contractions for a long time. They are very hard and can last quite a while. They increase as the uterus becomes more and more "irritable" (that's the official term). The childbirth classes, if you took them, ought to help you recognize when you're in labor. Basically, the contractions increase; gradually they become more frequent, painful, and regular. Check with your obstetrician about what signs to look for, and when to go to the hospital. Have him describe the "breaking of the water" and the "pink show" (or "bloody show"), since these usually signal the onset of labor. Find out what phone number you should use to call him. Then when you think you are in labor and you call, he'll tell you whether it's time to come to the hospital or not.

One nice thing about pregnancy lasting such a very long time is that you've really had your fill of it by the time you go into labor. You've been kicked long enough, you've really gotten the idea that the baby is not you, and you're probably uncomfortable enough that you wish it would just happen. Even if you are frightened about what labor is going to be like, you are probably so fed up with being pregnant and so curious to see *who* the heck the baby is, you're more impatient than afraid. You are ready!

Having that baby

When you, your husband, and your obstetrician decide that you must be in labor, rejoice! Feel like a shower? Why not? If it's your first baby, you probably have plenty of time, and somehow it seems terrific and improbable to take a shower when you think you're in labor. Then grab your suitcase and go. It's very exciting. It's like theater—dramatic, happening *now*, framed. It's happening to you, after all this long, long, long wait.

When you get to the hospital, you have to get checked in. Your husband has to park the car, and there are no spots. The cop tells him he has to find a proper place, so you get out of the car and go into the hospital alone. How mundane and unceremonious. How come they don't give proper weight to the fact that you and your husband are about to have your baby?

Inside, they seem uninterested that you are in labor. The fact is, they've seen it before, lots and lots. They all take their time, and it seems forever. They ask you to spell your name and things like that. Other women and men sit in their chairs, waiting their turns. Little suitcases sit beneath their knees. This scene doesn't fit your expectations! Didn't you imagine everyone rushing to prepare the bed, people scurrying, bustling—you know, like a hospital? You know, like on TV?

Here you are instead, stuck with a grumpy person who is telling you to follow her. If she *is* in a bad mood, don't take it personally. Also, let her know that you don't appreciate it.

They bring you to the prep room and someone examines you and asks you how frequent the contractions are, and they shave you, perhaps, and take your blood pressure. Now we're getting somewhere. But where is your husband? Can he find you? (He will.) You put on the awful hospital gown, and maybe you're shivering. It's good to bring socks because your feet get cold. They tell you to stuff your clothes in a bag they hand you. They put a hospital bracelet on you, and they prepare one for the baby! Now we're talking!

Miserably, you may notice that your contractions have slowed up a lot. Or maybe they seem to have gone away. This is an extremely common occurrence. Maybe the excitement of gearing up to come to the hospital, the car ride, and the check-in procedure have something to do with it. Whatever, it's disappointing that nothing seems to be happening anymore. Did you make a mistake and come in for nothing? Well, probably not. After a while, most likely, the contractions will start picking up again, and you're off and running. They've probably gotten you set up on a bed someplace, and maybe by now your husband is by your side, and you wait.

Waiting, again? This is probably the most passive time there is. Pretend you and your body are separate, and observe it if you can. Let your body have those contractions. There is nothing you can do about it. If you've learned breathing exercises, use them; they will keep you from interfering with the process of the contractions. Try to relax. Your husband can help a lot here by soothing and encouraging you, reassuring you that you're doing fine, and so on.

It may help to imagine that you are at the ocean, the waves are very strong, and you are body surfing. You see a big wave coming, you get ready, and you let it overtake you and overpower you. You concentrate on holding your breath in the water. You don't try to fight the waves because you know they are stronger than you. You let them take over and bring you to shore. You may be frightened because the waves are so powerful and sometimes come very fast, but you remind yourself that in a few seconds you will be past the tumult, you will be breathing normally, and you will be waiting for the next wave.

Coming in with the waves is a good analogy for labor insofar as it depicts a physically overpowering sensation. But labor is not romantic. And, unlike the waves at the beach, the contractions hurt. That's what makes it hard to relax. When you anticipate and worry about the next contraction, you get tense, and the tension exacerbates the pain. That's why you try to dissociate yourself from what's going on in your body so it can just happen—without you, almost. Remember that the contractions are opening up your cervix so the baby will be able to be born. Just go with it.

Labor is not sexual, either. Have you seen those books about childbirth with pictures of the laboring woman on the floor, naked and with long flowing hair, and surrounded by warm, supportive friends and family? Why is she naked? The implication of photos like these is that labor is sexual; if not, then why the naked breasts? If she's naked because her labor makes her hot and sweaty, then why isn't her hair tied back? These photos do a disservice to women who have not yet had a child. You get the idea that you're supposed to have a sexual experience in labor, and that if you don't like the idea of being surrounded by friends while you're laboring nakedly away, then you're an uptight prude. Labor is hard work. It hurts, it's tedious, it's impersonal, it's boring. You don't go into labor expecting orgasms.

It's not really possible to imagine labor before you go into it, and this fact can add to your anxiety beforehand. It's a relief to actually be in labor so you can dispense with the anticipation and get on with it. It's hard to accept the idea that labor can actually be boring, isn't it? But it is. A deck of cards and other games can help pass the time. You can joke with the doctors and nurses if you feel like it. Nurses, residents, your doctor, and whoever is on the floor all come in to check you, chat, listen to the baby's heartbeat, and so on. It drags. You take time out to have the contractions, and in between them you feel normal and can talk again and get back to the game. "Geography" is a good game for labor. Think of some others you like to play before you go into labor so you'll have some mechanism for getting through the boring parts, the tedium.

There's a momentum to labor, too, an acceleration. The contractions come faster and faster. It can be scary; sometimes you can barely catch your breath. Your husband or friend is there to reassure you, and this reassurance is very helpful now. You may feel out of control, and it is good to hang onto the rhythm of the breathing exercises. In a way it helps to consider yourself out of control from the beginning so that by now you are used to it. Let it take over. The doctor may ask you if you want something to help, and maybe you will. Demerol relaxes you enough so that you can rest in between the contractions, maybe even sleep. Check about the possible effects on the baby, which vary according to what stage of labor you're in. How are you doing? Decide on the basis of these considerations.

Then you finally find out that your cervix is dilated enough, and it is time to push. This part of labor can be quite exhilarating, and extremely hard work. You are pushing for all you are worth. Nurses and other personnel might be cheering you on, telling you what a good push that was, how strong you are, how well you're doing; they're getting you ready to be stronger still for the next one. Pu-sh-sh-h-h-h! The baby will be born soon! Maybe they move you into the delivery room now, or maybe you are in a birthing room where you get to stay put. Maybe, for whatever reason, you have to have a cesarean, but the main thing is you want to have this baby soon, and safely.

Amazement as the baby is born. Are you watching

in the mirror? The slimy creature comes out. It is incredible. There is a race to see who can tell the sex first. And it's announced! Maybe you already knew the sex from amniocentesis or from a sonogram, and this is a confirmation. Pretty exciting. The baby is born, it's a boy or a girl. You see the long, writhing umbilical cord; the cord gets cut; the baby gets cleaned up; the placenta is born; the obstetrician sews you up, perhaps; nurses massage your belly to stimulate your uterus to go back to shape. They put big sanitary pads on you. In between all this you hear some funny crying sounds. They weigh the baby, they examine him and give him Apgar scores, and finally *you* get to see him. Wow.

Maybe you have arranged with the obstetrician to have your husband participate fully in the delivery. That's special. It's terrific if he wants and is allowed to cut the umbilical cord. It's great if they lower the lights in the delivery room after the main work and cleaning up has been done. It's nice to hold the baby immediately, maybe nurse him.

What is it like holding your newborn? Now you know newborns don't look cute. It's okay if you think he's the ugliest thing you ever saw. You're going to have lots of conflicting emotions, and it's *all* all right. You'll probably change your mind over and over. How's your husband? Glowing? You're both exhausted and pretty exhilarated. It's over. You're a genius. You did it! It is a spectacular event.

After a while they bring you to your room. In some places you have to go to a recovery room first, but maybe instead the baby can stay with you, and the three of you can become acquainted a little bit. Maybe she's screaming. Maybe she's just looking around. You're counting toes and fingers, tracing your finger in the creases of her ears, touching her gingerly. She looks so delicate.

Okay, now let's move ahead a few hours. Your husband has made a lot of phone calls. Maybe he's gone home to sleep. You're resting. If you've had medications or anaesthetics, they are wearing off now. The nurses keep coming in to check you. They are checking your fundus (whatever that is). They want to make sure the uterus is contracting. They change the pads. They move you to and fro. The elevator is right next to your room, and it's noisy. They tell you your bladder is full. You can't tell. Everything down there feels strange, as if you don't know where it all is. Your tummy is still there. It's tender, chunky, and bumpy; it feels wrong. You thought it was going to be flat, right? It's not at all. You may feel very happy, or you may be surprised and disappointed that you feel awful. It's okay.

They put you on the bed pan. It's hard to go. Maybe the nurse runs the water in the sink. That helps. They tell you if you don't urinate soon, they will have to catheterize you. So you try to go, and maybe you do. Hooray. The bed pan is removed. What a relief. They change your bedding sixty million times. They keep the pads on you because you're bleeding, as if it's a huge menstrual period. Menstruation seems so long ago, but you remember. It's very nice to be in your room and not in the labor room. You remember that it's over; you have a son or daughter. You're a mother. Imagine! You're incredibly happy. You want to make some phone calls. You want to sleep. You're too excited to sleep. Maybe you hurt and ache. Can't get comfortable. Be patient. It will all get better, but it takes a while and it's good to recognize this *in advance*. Rest, if you can.

You notice that you're part of a bustling hospital routine. The meals will come. They'll keep changing and checking you, but less frequently. Eventually, you'll get up and explore what's different about your body. It still feels so strange. You go to the bathroom by yourself, maybe. The nurse shows you how to change the pads. You ask about taking a shower. You're a little woozy, perhaps. You'll have to go slowly at first. Your body hurts. You shuffle. Even if you've had no medication, you're still exhausted, spacy. And if you've had a cesarean, you're much more wiped out.

Visitors will come soon. What excitement. Visits tire you out incredibly. You want people to come, but at the same time it's too much. The loudspeaker is always going. Someone wants to know if you want to rent a TV. You're told to fill out a birth certificate. You're still deciding on names. The name you've picked doesn't seem to fit the baby you produced. Or maybe it does. They bring the baby. He's all wrapped up. It's time to nurse or give him the bottle. He's still not very hungry. He's precious and seems so strange. The nurse goes out of the room, and the baby's crying, and you're asking yourself what you're doing wrong, and when are you going to get the hang of it? Ask a friendly nurse to help.

Maybe it's hard to sleep. Should you take a sleeping pill if you're nursing? Your doctor will have an opinion on this. What about something for pain? Find out what's recommended. Getting some comfort and much-needed sleep may well be worth it, for you and the baby.

You'll probably be urged to attend a baby-bathing

instruction session given by one of the senior-looking nurses. There you all will sit, after shuffling protectively down the hall in fuzzy slippers to the nursery. There you will sit in pink bathrobes with weary, dull faces, and there you will watch the efficient nurse pluck a sample baby from among the ones you've produced and expertly wash hair, and deftly wipe discharges from neck creases, nose, ears, and eyes from nose-end out. You feel as if you should be taking notes, as if she'll be giving you a tough quiz at the end of this. Remember that you'll be out of her clutches soon, and she will be unable to check up on you at home, thank goodness.

You may be chafing at the bit to go home right away. You don't feel too bad, right? If the doctor thinks you're up to it, maybe you could go home very soon. But the main advantage of staying a little longer is that you will get some rest that you badly need even if some of the hospital routines irritate you.

Things are being taken care of for you here, but already you're getting a preview of the way it will be at home. Is your telephone ringing all the time, especially when you've decided to rest? It will do that at home, too. Maybe you'll decide to put the word out that you'll call them.

Also, you may have noticed that the timings of visitors, your meals, and the baby's meals conflict sometimes (or all the time). This is an excellent preview. Trying to figure out what to do is very confusing. In most if not all hospitals, visitors are not permitted in the room when the baby is there, but your hospital may be lax, and your friends may arrive during the baby's feeding. (And indeed, you may conspire for this to happen.) Now what do you do if they've brought you the baby, and then the food tray arrives, and then a visitor sneaks in, and then you have to go to the bathroom, and now the baby is crying (and you're starving)? Well, you can always ask a nurse to help. That is one of the great things about being in the hospital a few days. And you can also try to decide which things should come first and which things can wait. Something can always wait—even the baby.

What, the baby can wait?! Are you *allowed* to do that? Isn't this the beginning of terrible mothering, of cruel, callous behavior? No. One of the very difficult things about getting used to having a newborn is that there are a lot of conflicting things going on all at the same time, and you have to make choices. That's all.

This baby is pretty fantastic. What a creation! She's also quite scary. She may have a very loud, angry-sounding voice. It is natural that you don't know what to do. It is helpful to distinguish among the many nurses who are administering to you, find a few whom you like, and get help from them. Write all those dumb questions down, if it helps. Also, ask the pediatrician questions.

Now, how's your body doing? It needs attention, too. Is the obstetrician telling you that you have to have a bowel movement before you leave? This may be hard to do. Eventually, all these things will get easier, honest. How are your breasts? They may be quite engorged—full and hot and hard. They will feel better after a few days. Aspirin helps. If you are nursing, the hard feeling will be present off and on, depending on how often the baby nurses and other things. What about your nipples?

You need to take care of them. They may be tender from that baby, who, you are discovering, is quite strong. Thwock! he goes. When the baby latches on to nurse, what power! If your nipples hurt a lot, use the lanolin and ask for a nipple shield, which will protect the nipples while the baby nurses.

In other words, you'll be running into some problems here and there. You can get help with most if not all of them.

Coming home

It's very exciting to get ready to come home. Collect last-minute information and advice from the nurses you like, pack all your clothes, vases of flowers, chocolate, and other gifts, and try to rest until your husband, or friend, or relative comes to pick you up.

You have to get the baby ready. For the first time you put him in the clothes that *you* choose. Then there are papers to fill out so you can be discharged from the hospital, and pretty soon you're off.

Now you get home. If your husband has to rush back to work, I hope you have someone else there who can help you. If your mother is coming, I suggest that she get there before you so your lunch will be ready. Or, if your husband can stay, it's nice if he can make you your lunch. Just so you're not all of a sudden plunked down in your once-familiar habitat, which has now become strange with the addition of this new baby.

Everything is really different, you see. You have had a rite of passage; you have truly crossed into another world now with the birth of your baby. Nothing is the same. You have to relearn things, become reacquainted with things. It takes a while to figure out that *everything* is new, first of all; then it takes a while more before you can get used to it.

Maybe you put the baby in her crib, for starters. Doesn't she look tiny in there? Maybe you start to unpack all her things and your things. But it's tiring, hard work! You are probably very fatigued, and perhaps you cannot understand why you should be *this* tired. It's been a few days since you had the baby, and all you did was sit in the car on the way home, and you're *so* exhausted. It's very discouraging, but it's normal. You really are tired, and you should respect your tiredness rather than be disgusted with yourself for it.

Now is the time to take care of yourself, but good. If people are offering to help you, allow them to. You should let your husband, your mother, your mother-in-law, your sister, or whoever it is you've installed to help take over. You should try not to worry about the fact that your home is a mess, and don't concern yourself with meals and shopping. See if you can convince whoever is taking care of things to make as many decisions as possible without you. Being asked how you like your tomatoes sliced for the salad can be the straw that reduces you to hysterics. Your friend will be doing you a great favor if she buys her brand of cottage cheese rather than consulting you.

Are you nursing? You need to do two things in particular: make sure you're eating okay, and make sure you're getting some rest. These two things are necessary so you'll build up a proper milk supply. You're going to be getting up at night, maybe several times each night, and you may have trouble getting back to sleep. So whenever the baby is sleeping, you should try to get your rest. I know this is hard to do; when you are home, there are a lot of competing interests. You're used to being up and around. It was easy to rest in the hospital since there was nothing else to do, but now that you're home, it seems natural to get back to your routine. *Resist.*

Or maybe you want to talk with your mother, sister, whoever it is, since you haven't seen that person for so long. But try not to. Really, rest when the baby is sleeping. Try not to read; try not to write thank-you notes. Try to lie completely flat and close your eyes. It helps.

You won't always feel this wiped out. It's hard to imagine before you have the baby that you will feel this tired; and when you are this tired, it's hard to imagine that you will one day be rested again. But, you will. If you have had a cesarean, you will have to allow yourself more time to get back to normal. You've got major surgery to recover from on top of the normal adjustment to motherhood.

You may also feel blue. You can blame your hormones for that. They're a mess right now trying to readjust. And, furthermore, you've got a great deal of catching up to do emotionally. It's a big deal to have a baby, and it takes a while for your system to recognize it. Here the passive rule applies again; you can only do so much to speed up the process. It takes time. Just how long depends on who you are, what kind of temperament you have, how you adapt to changes normally, and all kinds of other things. Maybe you'll get right into the swing of things because you happen to live in a neighborhood with many young mothers with infant children, you have known the other mothers for years, they have been with you all through your pregnancy, and they are ready and eager to support you now. Lucky you! Even so, it will take several weeks, at least. But maybe you don't know many people near you, and you haven't seen any infants around. You feel isolated —except at the moment, when you are surrounded by noisy, excited, laughing family. It seems to be all extremes.

If you've had a cesarean, you may feel very disappointed that the birth didn't go the "normal" way. You ought not to feel that way, but if you do, you do. Unless you've known ahead of time, you never expect a cesarean to happen to *you*. You might need some special understanding and time. Let yourself have it.

How quickly you recover will also depend on how you and your husband handle the big change of having a baby in your lives. No matter how well the two of you get along, you have a lot of negotiating and compromising to do, and a lot of exploring of how you each feel about everything. You are both in a brand-new situation for which you have no ready-made routines. It's all got to get worked out slowly. When the baby cries, for example, who picks him up, and after how long? Maybe you pick him up right away, but then you resent that your husband doesn't seem to be doing that enough. He tells you that you pick the baby up before he has a chance to, but you've been waiting as long as you can stand it. This is the kind of thing that has to get worked out, little by little. Maybe you can learn to stand the crying for an extra few seconds until he picks the baby up, and maybe he can learn to pick the baby up a little quicker. That's where the good will of your relationship comes into play.

The ease of the adjustment the two of you make also depends on the particular baby you end up with. The baby may be only four days old now, but believe it or not, you both know a great deal about this child already. She was born with a particular temperament to begin with, and you have already noticed that she has a particularly harsh, shrill scream, or that she is docile and quiet and sleeps a lot. Many of the qualities you notice now are part of the personality she was born with (and which you and she are stuck with).

I'm not diminishing the importance of environment when I say this. However, I am challenging the birth-order hypothesis, which is reigning dominant these days. People will tell you that first-born children are difficult because the parents are tense. The second kids are easygoing, the birth-order hypothesis continues, and it's much easier for everyone because the parents have been through it once before. This is simplistic thinking. It assumes that the way the baby behaves depends entirely on her environment—on the way you behave, her position in the family, and other particulars of her upbringing. But it leaves out of the equation entirely what the kid brings to the situation—her temperament, specifically. You have produced a person who is new, and who will be influenced tremendously by the world around her. But there is a lot that came ready-made in this child, and *you* are going to have to adapt to it. And you have only begun to know her.

Anyhow, all these things will determine how quickly things get back to normal. Or, I should say, how quickly they get back to a *new* normal.

The first week or so

What's going on at your home these first days? How many relatives are there? Is it very noisy or very quiet? Has your husband gone back to work, or is he at home with you? Do you feel lonely, besieged, both, neither? Of course, this all varies immensely, depending on your particular situation. Maybe you live near your relatives, and you are used to seeing them all the time, and they are around a lot now, and it doesn't seem very different from usual. But maybe your parents flew in from the other coast, and this visit is special. You've saved up many things to tell one another, and if you feel any irritation, you mustn't let it show. It's tricky when you've got relatives whom you haven't seen for ages; it takes so long to get things flowing easily again between you, and it's a strain having to work to achieve that interaction again. It's especially tricky if you don't get along very well with them normally.

No matter what, whether it's easy between all of you or not, it's a good idea to make sure *you* take off here and there to lie down all by yourself and take a breather. This is doubly important if you've got other kids. Then the activity and the jabbering and everything that's going on between the kids and their grandparents, aunts and uncles, and so forth, is so lively and stimulating that you've got to protect yourself and go underground. At these times you may feel that you're never going to make it. If it's bothering you so much, you wonder, what are you doing having kids? Why on earth did you ever think you were cut out for this? How can you turn the clock back and reverse the decision? How *could* you have ever been so wrong about anything?

Go lie down, whether you are thinking these frightening thoughts or not. Little by little, some of your tension eases, like a headache reluctantly relinquishing its grip. You need to rest. You need to have people nearby, but you also need to be by yourself with real quiet. In fact, you need some conflicting things. You need advice, and you need to find things out by yourself. You need to be with the baby, and you need to be away from the baby. You need to have contact with your friends, but the visits and phone calls tire you out. The right amounts and proportions of these things vary, so you have to feel it all out, little by little.

The baby—what's happening with the baby? Did you just decide to take a nap, and you hear the baby crying? Are they going to pick him up or not? Do you think he's hungry again, *already*? You check your baby manual. It says the baby has growth spurts. Is this a growth spurt? Let's say you're nursing. You're still building up your milk supply. That poor baby is *so* hungry, you imagine, and you don't have enough milk. Maybe you should feed him again, even though you just finished, because it will stimulate more milk production and, besides, the nursing is soothing to him. After all, he was just born and is newly home, and there are lots of noises around, and he's not used to his crib, and a zillion things could be bothering him. *And you don't know what they are!* But don't forget, your doctor suggested that you shouldn't nurse too often because it will tire you out, and being tired reduces the milk supply. Nothing like Catch-22, huh? But the baby kept falling asleep the last time you nursed him, and maybe he didn't get enough. Maybe now he's really hungry. But now you're frazzled, and your mother is asking what you want to do about the baby, dear, and you really don't want to nurse again (and your nipples may be sore), but maybe you should, and *you just don't know!*

Well, how can you know? The baby is tiny. He's just been born, and his system is adjusting as fast as it can, but not fast enough. Lots of things happening in his body just aren't finished yet. His nerves are busy myelinating; his digestive system is full of kinks. He's busy getting used to sounds, lights, the taste of milk, the feel of your skin, the feel of clothes, the changing temperatures; so many things are happening. The baby is probably having a harder time of it than you are (though at least he's less conscious of it than you are, and it's easier for him to be passive). The most you can do is try to make him more comfortable. If he keeps on crying and you can't figure out anything else to do, then close his door, or hold him, or give him to your mother-in-law to hold—whatever bothers you the least. And get back to your nap.

It's dinner time. The baby's not due to be fed for another hour or so; your mother has fixed up a fine dinner; and all of you are sitting down to eat. Ears prick up. The unmistakable sounds of a baby crying reach the table. You burst into tears. It's not time; it's not fair. What's the *matter* with him? You and your husband look sadly at each other. Then, resolutely, you both start to eat. The hell with the baby!

But your mother wants to see what the matter is. She wants to do what she can. She looks for your permission to go pick him up. You wish she wouldn't. You were all going to sit down to supper without that kid interrupting the *second* you began.

Now I'll tell you what would improve this situation. You're all sitting down, forks in hand; the baby cries; you and your husband moan; and then the other relatives, parents, in-laws, whoever—all the grown-ups —join you in feeling outraged about your totally obnoxious baby. The point is, you and your husband are the ones who need the allies, not the baby. One of the grown-ups should not be defecting to the camp of the baby at this moment. This is the time to join in unison in resisting that child. *Then* one of you can get the baby. Maybe he just wants to sit in the infant seat and watch you all.

Have your parents become new grandparents with

the birth of your child? They have adjustments to make, too. You don't know what it all means to them yet, and they don't either. Maybe they have been bugging you for years to provide them with a sweet grandchild, but maybe now that it's happened, they're not so sure they like all the cultural connotations of grandparenthood. (Do they really like it when their friends call them Grandpa and Grandma?) Maybe they weren't at all anxious for you to have kids and make them grandparents, and they feel too young for all this. Does this birth, and the change of status for them, make them "old"? How should they behave towards you now that you are a parent? How many "rights" do they have in relation to their grandchild, your child?

Maybe your parents don't want to be considered ready-made babysitters for you. Maybe they're somewhat worried that you're going to relegate them to the status of doddering grandparents. Maybe they won't want to be always regaled with stories about your beautiful child when she gets a tooth or learns to sit up.

Conflicting and complicated feelings are involved. Your child may remind your parents of you in your infancy, and this may make them feel buoyant, wistful, remorseful, strangely young, intolerably old. They may want to talk about their memories of you, and when you react impatiently, they may feel rebuffed and hurt. They're *experts*, after all, but they know you have to learn it all yourself—just as when you were a kid and didn't want to wear a jacket when it was freezing out. And even though they're experts, and can feel the memory of you as a baby in their arms somewhere, so much of it has escaped that they can't grasp it to express it to you. They see you glowing with your child, and they recognize your feeling that your baby is unique, wonderful, and full of promise. They remember feeling that way, and they know, too, the disappointments of seeing where and how the infinite potential of the newborn becomes limited. Their wise summations, their assurances that "this too shall pass," may irritate you incredibly. For them this baby eclipses time, and stretches it out endlessly between you as well. They feel close to you now that you are a parent like them, and at the same time they feel more distant from you than ever.

Just like you and your child, the grandparents are unique. They respond to your new baby in their own ways, and they, too, undergo an evolving process as they get used to being grandparents, having a grandchild, and seeing their child become a parent. They, too, will need time.

The entrance of a baby into your lives changes everyone in a kind of ripple effect. The new individual who has been introduced into your world modifies the old interactions. New patterns of getting along must be developed, and in the meantime they are all under negotiation and the stress of change. That's why there is no right way to do any of this. The solutions are novel and different for everyone.

Now, what's happening with the nursing? You and the baby are trying to figure it all out. You may be worried that the baby is not getting enough, or getting too much. (Why is she spitting up so much?) You may think you must be doing something very wrong since she cries sometimes while she is nursing. You may be afraid that you are tense and that the baby is sensing it, and that your terrible emotional state is wrecking things.

Passive time. Sometimes the baby cries no matter what you do, because of and despite everything. So when you are nursing the baby, get comfortable, maybe have a beer, be by yourself if you want, and let the baby have a go at it. If the baby is crying, it's not your fault. It's not her fault, either. The baby is going to have to cry quite a bit before things get right. She has a hard time keeping hold of the nipple, or finding it; the milk doesn't come fast enough, then it comes too fast; then she chokes and coughs, and because she gets upset and starts crying, she's too wound up to get back to nursing again. What do you do in the meantime? Maybe you can talk to her gently, soothingly; maybe you can pat her, burp her. But maybe, whatever you do, she still doesn't settle down, and the two of you are getting nowhere (and the beer isn't helping). At this point I suggest you put her back in her crib. She will fall asleep or she won't. You'll know soon enough. You take a short break in the meantime; go tell your mother what a creepy baby you have and how you wish she'd never been born. Go to the bathroom; finish your beer; look at the front page of the paper. Now—is she still crying? Maybe if she is you can try again. Maybe she burps. Hooray! Maybe the two of you settle down again, and the nursing goes a little better. Maybe you're just a tiny bit more patient now that you've been away for a few minutes, and maybe her fussing doesn't get to you quite as much as it did a while before.

You just may have a baby who cries a lot, and it may not have anything whatever to do with you. The baby may be colicky, and the milk may be hard to digest. Colic happens with breast-fed babies, too, you know (and with second-born children, and with relaxed mothers!). But whether you have a colicky baby or not, he's probably getting plenty of milk, and he's probably growing just fine.

Did people tell you how you'd "bounce back" in a week or so? They didn't bounce back themselves, you know, but they thought maybe you would, and they mistakenly thought you'd be jubilant to have their vote of confidence. But *no one* bounces back right away. It takes time for everyone, lots of time. In the meantime, trust yourself.

More jumbled feelings

It really *is* different from what you expected, isn't it? Didn't you think you'd be filled with relief and happiness once the baby was born? And now you're not? It will get better. (Don't you believe me?) I've been describing the postpartum scene in detail to make concrete the mixed-up, bewildering array of things that go on after you have a baby. The pettiness of having a baby is totally beyond belief before you have one. This overwhelming pettiness is intertwined with your exploding emotions. That's something that you probably never expected beforehand. Before getting pregnant you were probably used to keeping your tasks and your emotions mostly separate. Now, they are completely joined. It's hard. It's exhausting.

Are you worried about the baby all the time? When he's sleeping do you wonder why he's sleeping so long? One nice thing about having the baby outside of you is that when you are worried, you can just go check on him. That's very reassuring. And you do it a lot. You need the constant reassurance that he's really breathing, really alive. After all, you're not feeling the kicking inside you anymore.

Though the baby seems to be all right, do you have the vague feeling you're doing something wrong? Does he eat at 1:30, 4:00, 5:50, and 10:20 rather than at 2:00, 6:00, and 10:00, as the book says? You wonder when you and he will get on the "right" schedule that you've read about.

You're angry, too. You want your body back to yourself, but if you're nursing, your child still claims it. He spits up on you, and he grabs your hair. You're the center of things, but you're not. Everyone leaves you alone, or they don't. You're angry at yourself, perhaps, for not feeling the way you thought you would feel. You may be angry that so much seems out of control, beyond your abilities, and unlike your expectations.

You feel as if you're the only woman on earth to have actually produced a baby! No one ever really did it before. Each woman somehow has to rediscover how it's done since so much of that knowledge is incommunicable. Coupled with the feeling of being a genius for having carried it off is the awareness, which grows over weeks and months, of how absolutely mundane having a baby is. When you finally venture out of the house to go to the store, and you see a mother with a year-old child, you wonder how she ever survived. And you catch yourself sounding like a ridiculous expert—talking about your baby all the time as if no one has ever had one before.

Something else, too. Now that you are a mother, you think about your own mother in a new way. She *must* have had some of the same experiences, some of the same feelings that you are having. Now, maybe for the first time in your life, it grabs you that she was once the same age you are right now. She all of a sudden becomes a little more understandable. She too knew little; she too worried a lot; maybe she even felt as alone as you do. Maybe you feel closer to her now.

This makes you think about yourself as the mother of this child. There are many things the baby will never understand about *you*. Until maybe one day when *she* has a baby. The generation gap is always opening and closing, unendingly.

And one more thing—if your mother was once your age, then you can one day be her age. This means that you participate in the aging process. You will one day get old. Having a baby means coming to understand that you are included in this scheme. This knowledge never faced you so starkly before. Oh well—now you can forget it.

What's a mother supposed to be, anyway?

You've all of a sudden become a mother, but you're still a kid and you know it. Do you hide this from everyone? How does a person make the emotional transition to motherhood? You already know it's not automatic; you've been waiting around for it to hit you over the head, and it hasn't. When will it happen, and what does it entail?

First of all, you can stay who you are. A big shift has occurred: you and your husband have produced a baby, and you and he are now completely responsible for this new, little organism. But you don't have to drop everything now and become a faceless, giving, spongy, milk machine named Mom. You stay who you are. To do so, however, you have to fight.

When you were pregnant, you learned that the fetus was a separate being. This got you into practice looking out for yourself at the same time that the child was getting her nourishment. You have to keep looking out for yourself.

Just because you have become a mother doesn't mean you don't have choices. You don't have to just stop everything and wait for the baby to call all the shots. New mothers need practice in learning when the babies come first, and when they don't. Mothers need help in defining themselves vis-à-vis the imperious infants. They need to do this right from the start so that they teach themselves and their children that they have rights, too. They need to learn it's even all right that they don't like their children every minute.

The baby is one week old. You've had a terrible night. You fed him at 10:30, then at midnight, then at 2:00 AM, then at 5:00. But after the 5:00 AM nursing he kept crying off and on. Your husband walked him for a while, and then you did. You wondered about nursing him again, but he finally fell back to sleep. But then you were so mad and frustrated, you couldn't go back to sleep yourself. Now it is 7:30, and your mother wants to fix you an egg for breakfast. You tell her to forget it. Everything is terrible; you just know that as soon as you start to eat, the baby will wake up to be fed again. Your mother convinces you anyhow, and you reluctantly agree.

You pick up the fork to start eating the egg, and, wouldn't you know, the baby is crying. And so are you. You start to get up, totally defeated again. But your mother stops you. "Wait," she says. "Eat that egg! You need to eat first. The baby will outlive you, you know."

You need to hear this. You and the baby are separate. The baby's needs do not diminish yours. You must not let them. You are the one who has to have strength so that you will be able to mother that child, and withstand him sometimes, too.

Of course the baby has overwhelming needs. You're not forgetting that—how can you with him crying all the time? But you're exhausted and achy; you need time alone, need to get things straight, and need to be with your husband.

The baby manuals that you have geared yourself with are teaching you how to fulfill your baby. You can create the smartest kid in town if you make your own toys, grind your own food, change all your eating habits, throw out the television, and so on. But you will also be participating in the myth that the baby's environment totally determines how she will turn out, and furthermore, you will be teaching the baby that she is the center of the universe.

I don't think you should teach your baby that the world begins and ends with her. You shouldn't do it for anybody's sake, and certainly not yours. You're going to be getting books about how to discipline the child later on, and you're going to be reading all about limiting this and that. Well, you have to get into practice. You don't just start disciplining the baby's appetite for everything at one year, eight months, and twenty-three days. You start in the beginning by simply taking you and your husband into account. The baby has needs; you and your husband have needs. The hard work is to make them mesh, more or less. You don't just go and subjugate all your needs to the baby's.

What this means is that when all hell is breaking

loose, the phone is ringing, the baby is crying, and you are on the toilet worrying about your hemorrhoids, you don't drop everything and get the baby. Stay where you are! Even though you've read the book that says when the baby is three months old you should be sure to pick him up when he cries so he learns to trust. Not if it means hemorrhoids, you don't! So what if he doesn't trust you implicitly forever after that. It's good practice for him. (He'll learn people aren't completely trustworthy sooner or later anyhow.)

It means that you do nice things for yourself here and there. You have a drink at the neighbors, even though you're nursing, because it makes you feel like you're an adult; you're an autonomous person with a valid ID. You quit nursing at three months rather than at six because it doesn't thrill you, and you feel too tied down. So what about all the antibodies the baby doesn't get! If you need to stop, stop.

You and your husband manage to get away from the baby overnight, or for a weekend, and you give yourself the privilege of not feeling guilty that you don't miss her. Why should you miss her? You've sure seen enough of her.

In other words, you respect yourself enough to give yourself some time. You value your marriage enough to give it some consideration. Make time for yourself little by little (it's not easy), and you start to get the idea, and the baby does, too. Both you and the child need the *daily* practice of learning that you are a separate individual. Then, when you want your five-year-old to stop jabbering while you're reading the paper, you'll already have established some precedent.

Right from the start with that sweet, tiny, ferti-
lized egg nestled comfortably inside you, it and you
were separate *and* linked. This relationship continues
with the balance between separateness and closeness
shifting all the time. Your child will want to confide in
you and cling to you, and she will have secrets and will
shut the door to her bedroom on you. And so it goes.
Her shyness will remind you of yourself, but her math-
ematical prowess will shock you with the realization
that she's not your clone.

Whether you go back to paid work or not, mothering is a real occupation, a legitimate job. If you elect to
"devote" yourself to mothering, you still have parts of
yourself that are separate, and you still have other roles.
As a mother you command respect, from your child as
well as from everyone else.

Advice revisited

Sometimes other people can really mess you up. Here you are, struggling along with your baby; you and your husband are both sleep-deprived, bleary-eyed, confused, frazzled. You don't know which end is up, but when you try to analyze the situation, it seems as if having a new baby in the house shouldn't be *this* disruptive, this difficult, and this perplexing. Yet, it is—there's just no getting around that. And right along with all your doubts, fears, and fatigue comes unsolicited advice and admonitions from everyone.

"What?!" they exclaim. "He's not sleeping through the night *yet*? Are you sure you have enough milk? I started my Joey on cereal when he was two weeks old, and he was sleeping through right away." Or you hear this: "Of course, you're nursing her on demand, right?" Or this: "Never feed your baby whenever she wants it, or she'll never extend the time between feedings!" Not to mention: "The best thing is to nurse the baby lying down; it's so relaxing," along with: "Always feed the baby in an upright position so the bubbles have a chance to come up," plus: "The baby will be dependent and will always want to sleep with you if you let him get used to your nursing him in bed."

Help! If you thought the opinions you got while you were pregnant were vociferous, conflicting, and confusing, the comments you hear now are more so. They cover the gamut—how to feed the baby, when to take the baby outside, how much weight the baby should gain, when to introduce solid foods, when the baby should wear shoes, when you and your husband should resume sex, how to treat the siblings, whether siblings should be given gifts when the new baby gets one, and so on ad infinitum.

You tell someone that you think your baby is colicky. You immediately get a sympathetic response; the other person knows how rough it can be, how terribly jarring the constant crying is. But right away come the suggestions, and they can be both troubling and helpful. "Ignore the crying," someone suggests (ruthlessly, you think, with admiration). "Comfort the baby, or she'll cry more to get you to respond next time," warns another.

Should you pick the baby up every time she cries? Should you let your jealous four-year-old be with you when you feed the baby, or should she be taught right away that the baby has to have some special time, too? Should you take the baby outside if it's cold? Do you have to give the baby a bath every day? Is the baby okay? How do you know? Really, there are no right answers. Almost always, it's a matter of feeling it out.

One thing about kids, too, is that something works with them one time, but then it doesn't work the next. It seems you are always busy trying to catch up. They are growing and changing so fast that you are always two steps behind them. That's why it doesn't make sense to listen to too much advice. The advice you get assumes that kids are the same, and that they are consistent. Neither is true. If something works for you, do it.

The principle here is twofold. A lot of things are going on. You have to take care of yourself and your own concerns; that's one thing. The other thing is that you are learning who your baby is. He is not the same kid whom the Higalo's had ten years ago. You may have a baby who really doesn't like to be handled much, but who loves funny sounds and enjoys being talked to and stroked gently. Or his mood may vary; one time he loves being held, and another time he's too fussy. You have to be receptive enough to let your child teach you who he is. You can't know ahead of time; you must continually learn.

By the same token, you are teaching your baby who you are. You don't have to be everyone and everything to your baby—you *can't* be. You've got your own personality and idiosyncracies, which are a combination of strengths and limitations, and your baby is learning how to deal with all of you. In a sense, then, your baby is learning about the real world through experiencing her caretakers. You're not perfect, and the baby will figure that out very soon. She'll learn to make allowances for you, learn to get around you, learn to love you, and so on. In other words, it's important to be yourself, both for yourself and the others close to you, and for the baby.

Some of your concerns are petty, and some of them are important. One of the difficult things about getting used to a baby is learning to distinguish the two. Your worries sort themselves out little by little, but in the beginning the petty things drive you nuts, and they are all mixed up with the important things. It's therefore natural to want advice and help, but you should pick your advice-givers carefully. If you are close to your mother, neighbor, or friend, and you trust her judgment, then that person is a good bet.

Another good advice-giver may be the pediatrician. Many pediatricians have hours during which you can call them with all the minor and major questions that have been plaguing you. The doctor might have her calling time from 7:30 to 8:30 in the morning at her home. You make a list of your questions: when can I introduce a supplementary bottle of formula? Is a rectal temperature of 102 degrees an emergency? She spit up a quart this morning! What should I do? How come the umbilicus smells? Why won't she stop crying? My mother says to bundle her up, but she looks so hot. And so on. Note your baby's age, and start your conversation with that information. If you can just get over feeling foolish about calling, you will probably feel better afterwards.

Otherwise, you and your husband make up your own minds about everything. Work it out between you. Find out each other's instincts and inclinations about the baby. Do what seems sensible; it probably is. Help the baby out, but respect yourselves, too. If you are generally nice people with good intentions, and you have the guts (and I mean *guts*) to trust yourselves, it'll probably work out fine.

Advice is of two distinct kinds. One kind is genuinely helpful. It comes from people who have listened—really listened—to what you're asking and what you're going through. Their advice, a bona fide response to that listening, can be extremely helpful, mainly because it takes you and your specific situation into account.

The other kind of advice is very different. The advice-giver has heard it all before. He knows ahead of time what you're going to say; he knows "that kind" of baby. The so-called advice from a person like this is pat, formulaic, competitive, and predictive. It is not helpful at all. It's often a put-down.

It's very important to know into which camp the information you are receiving falls. "Just you wait" is a signal to turn off. The person is assuming you are going to have the same experience she did. Her children are two years older than yours, and that gives her the license to generalize her experience to everyone, at least to you. Don't fall for it. She is talking only—I stress *only*—about herself. Remember that you are a different person and that you have a different child. It's a new ball game.

The first few weeks are such a mixed-up time. You are excited that you have a baby, of course, but your excitement is so intertwined with the confusion, the dismay, the anger caused by so much being difficult that you can barely acknowledge all your feelings to yourself. When feeding the baby goes well, you are filled with love for your child, but when it goes badly, you frighten yourself with fantasies of throwing him in the diaper pail. Then someone comes to visit, looks endearingly at the baby, at you, and at the beautiful picture you must make, and says wistfully, "If only they stayed like that . . ."

What! This is about the worst thing anyone could say. A comment like that implies that it gets worse, and that this time of total infant dependency is pure bliss for mother and child. You are a madonna with child; the lace curls around the two of you in an oval frame. You lovingly stroke her soft skin as she holds your finger and gazes adoringly into your face.

That's the way it's supposed to be, right? You've got the one kid in the world who screams bloody murder while nursing. You're the one mother in the world who hates her child and has no maternal instincts. Forget it.

The long and the short of it is that there are some wonderful things about total infant dependency, and there are some awful, miserable things about it. It's quite nice, at times, that there is so much you can and must do for your child, but it sure is a drag, too! Parents who wish children stayed like "that" are revising history, inventing their own experience of those first few months. They are talking wistfully about themselves, not about you and your baby.

Nonetheless, these kinds of things are very hard to hear. They don't stop, either. You just get better (and you will) at distinguishing them for what they are. At the same time you and your husband learn the ropes, and you learn that your own instincts are the best guide. Meanwhile you will be subject to advice in all different forms.

You tell your neighbor how your children seem to be teaching themselves higher math by constantly comparing to see who has more and who's getting cheated, and the neighbor knowingly utters, "It gets worse," never even noticing you've made a joke. In this way you determine who is and who is not a good audience for your humor.

When you are traveling with your three-month-old, it's been hell in the car, and someone says, "Now is the time to get all your traveling in because it becomes impossible later," tell yourself that that person can go jump in the lake. When you decide to have another baby and people tell you that two kids are more than twice one kid (got that?), remind yourself that they are talking about their own experiences. When your baby screams and they invite you to listen to their tales of the tantrums of "the terrible twos," *don't* take it literally. Just don't.

Another deus ex machina pronouncement is the gentle and infuriating saying, "Little children, little problems; big children, big problems." You'll jump off that bridge when you get to it, right? Do they have to tell you these things now?

In all these tales there is truth and distortion. A lot can be generalized about kids and bringing them up, but a lot can't be. It may be worth having a bunch of kids just so people stop giving you this kind of advice.

There are trade-offs at every age. Traveling with a

three-month-old is easier *in some ways* than traveling with a two-year-old. But in other ways taking trips with the two-year-old is much easier. The child understands language, can sometimes be reasoned with, and is often happy to be distracted because her interests are not restricted to basic physiological ones anymore. "The terrible twos" supposedly describes the nasty tantrums of ego-finding two-year-olds who want their own way. It's true that a lot of kids that age have tantrums, but again, it varies. Some of them fly off the wall; some are quite reasonable. Lots of parents wait around day after day for their kids to get into the "terrible twos," and it never happens. Those who talk about the "terrible twos" gloss over the fact that two-year-olds can be delightful in their discovery of selfhood. They are thrilled with it, and it's fun to watch them become self-sufficient and proud of themselves. So, it's a trade-off.

Having two kids can be harder than having one, but there's probably nothing harder than getting used to having a baby in the first place. With two, there are different kinds of problems and tasks. Five-year-olds may talk back to you, trick you, harass the new baby, and want you to take them to their friends' houses all the time, but they also can pick up their toys, entertain the new baby, and get a peach or carrot for themselves when they're hungry. It's all just too complex to sum up in the pat generalizations and warnings that you hear from everyone. So don't be scared off.

Why four weeks
is the worst

Here you are, four weeks postpartum. Things should be getting back to normal!

Afraid not. Four weeks, six weeks, or sometime around the first two or three months is about the worst. You're thinking that this is the way it's always, always, always going to be, and that it's never going to get better. You are fat. You are extremely tired all the time. You limp around still favoring the stitches. Your husband can't wait to have sex, and you want to, but you're afraid, and you're hoping the doctor will tell you that you shouldn't for the next six months. You're still bleeding, and you're worried that something is wrong. Your worry is vague, not big enough to call the doctor, but not small enough that it doesn't nag at you persistently. Your breasts leak all the time. Every time you feed the baby, he spits up all over you; you change your clothes, and then he does it again. You feel defeated by everything. And if you've had a cesarean, it's harder still, and takes longer. The good news is that all this doesn't get *worse*.

Very deep down you really believe that it's not going to get any better. You are convinced that you will always be this tired, this heavy, this dull, this weepy, this confused. You have no perspective, and that makes it so much worse. If you could only believe it will get better—that you'll get through it, that it just takes time, and that you will emerge again—it would make all the difference. But when you feel this blue you also lack that necessary perspective.

A note here about professional help. Though a certain amount of feeling blue is normal and just takes time to get over, you may feel uncomfortable enough that you should consider therapy. My descriptions of the postpartum time are meant to convey some of the difficulties of the transition to parenthood in a vivid way so that if you experience some of these difficulties, it won't be such a shock. But always consider talking to a professional if you think your unhappiness is excessive. Don't you deserve all the help you can get after what you've been through?

The baby gifts pile up. You've got thank-you notes to write, and you don't feel like writing them. The baby clothes are adorable, but you have the strength only to put the baby in undershirts, because putting on the clothes is such an ordeal, and they have to be changed so often. Your mental picture of taking nature walks with your newborn in his cozy new front-pack contrasts rudely with the difficulty of putting him in it, and his squirmy protest of it after he's installed. Everyone else's babies love having their limbs twisted into these things, of course.

Every time you start to do something the baby cries, and you don't know what it is this time. It's been only forty-five minutes since you last fed her. You're at home all by yourself; it was a relief when your mother (sister, mother-in-law, friend) went home, but you wish she were back. You want to crawl under a rock and hide, but you wonder where all your friends have gone. (They're probably afraid to "bother" you.) It is the pits.

Your husband comes home and asks you how it went today, and he looks a little dismayed when you tell him, but he doesn't really understand. You try to give him a minute-by-minute account, but he grows impatient and reminds you that he had frustrations and hard work today, too. You can't get across just *why* it's so hard. It's intangible.

It has to do with the fact that you're not in charge of your life anymore. The baby is tiny, but he controls the roost, it seems. You feel so incompetent that you can't get anything done, but you can't. You have implicit expectations that don't get fulfilled. For example, the baby slept for two hours. The whole time he slept, you kept listening and waiting for him to wake up. You were going to lie down while he napped, but since he slept for only fifteen minutes at the same time yesterday, you thought that was going to happen again today. So you kept doing little things around the place. You didn't want to start anything large, because you knew the baby would interrupt you, *but he didn't!*

Your expectations never get fulfilled. How can he do this to you? You go nuts.

It's not just, and it's not logical. When you understand this you're better off. (It usually takes a couple of kids.) What you have to learn to do is grab time whenever you can because you never know when your time is going to be grabbed back from you. You don't plan very much. Little by little (and it takes time) you learn to do things in snatches. You start to write the letter to your sister; the baby cries, so you write a little more, wondering if the baby will stop or not. When the baby keeps crying, you go to her and leave the letter. After you find that she's happy in the infant seat, you do the morning dishes, then go back to the letter. The baby starts squirming and crying in the infant seat. Now you decide it's time to feed her, so you do that, and you read a bit of the paper while you're at it. Finally, she's back in the crib, and you start picking up diapers, washing bottles, getting some lunch ready for yourself, and you then settle down to your letter, and she cries again.

That's the way it is. Some babies are predictable, but it always seems it's the other people who have them. You just aren't used to having to cater to someone else like this, and it's awful sometimes! But what have you done all day? You can't describe it; it's too chopped up, ragged, vague.

It's an ordeal to go anywhere. You want to go to the bank and then buy some avocados, but you don't want to do it now because it's only a half-hour until you're due to nurse the baby, so he'll probably be screaming the whole time. How do you time anything, and how do you fit things in?

Little by little, you just learn how. You learn how to put the baby in the car seat; you learn how to wake him up in the middle of a nap to go someplace; you learn how to carry a few things with you for contingencies; and you learn how to tune out some (and only some) of the crying when the whole big plan fails. In the meantime, you have to remember that your particular, difficult experience is very common. Especially common is the isolation and despondency that you feel. You imagine that all new mothers get back to doing things by now, and that since you're not, you never will be.

Talking about it helps a lot. Talk about it with your husband, and with the people you like. Get into therapy if it seems warranted.

When someone asks you how you are, tell them how awful it is. The shock of this kind of response will make it seem funny all of a sudden. When you tell women who have kids it's awful, you'll get instant recognition from them. They really know what you mean, but they'd never confided to you their own real feelings before.

You know why? Because when they went through it, they thought the awfulness was because of their own failings. They thought their colicky baby was screaming because of their tension, their bad mothering. They thought they were supposed to be bouncing back by now, but they weren't, and they never dreamed other women felt the same way. They thought it was their own fault. And when they finally recovered, and things got better, they forgot parts of it, were too ashamed to talk about the parts they remembered, and didn't want to tell you about it when you were pregnant because they didn't want to scare you. Besides, you'd probably be like all the other women they imagined who bounce right back.

It takes *time*, dammit. You can push yourself some

—to get out, to put on perfume, to get a babysitter—
but you can't do it all. Your husband should be sympathetic and available. It is hard, and while it is hard
for him, too, it's harder for you. Get all the help you
can get. You have to go easy on yourself and not expect
too much too soon. Slowly, little by little, you get there.

Pettiness
and the limits of control

For people used to getting work done, the jobs involved in tending a baby are frustrating simply because they are very repetitive and never complete. You wash the bottle right after she's through with it, not because it'll be washed and done with, but because the next time she's desperate for it you'll have it ready. You do the jobs you have to do so that you don't have three things to do in the space of one second.

Maybe a way to elevate these essentially mundane and mindless tasks is to think of yourself as the grease and the glue. The little things you keep doing—remembering to take the teething bisquits on the car ride, making sure the cup is washed out and ready—keep things meshing and prevent them from falling apart. They are essential in maintaining some harmony.

Shortcuts sometimes work, and sometimes they exacerbate the problems. You are wary about filling your two-year-old's juice cup because he might spill it, but he downs it expertly and insists on more. The routine repeats itself several times. Finally you calculate that a fuller cup will yield you an extra minute to eat your lunch. Natch, he spills it all over the table and the newspaper you're reading. Not only are you supposed to suppress your anger at him for having spilled the juice, but don't forget, he's still thirsty, and you need to pour him more.

The day when you put the garbage in the freezer, you know you've arrived. You make lists and you lose the lists. Remembering to give the children their vitamins every day seems impossible. There's always a great deal to do.

Just as in pregnancy, there are limits to your control over the process of parenting. When you go next door to welcome the new neighbors to town, your child immediately draws a picture in the fog from his breath on their gorgeous sliding glass doors. How could you possibly have stopped that in time? You hand the baby to your favorite uncle, and she throws up on him.

You have banned violent toys in your home, but that doesn't prevent your kids' chewing the toast into the shape of guns, does it? The hardest thing about recognizing your limits, I think, is that it forces you to change your image of yourself. Maybe you thought that *your* children would never fight with each other because you would love them well enough. Now they fight, and they fight, and they fight as if they really hate each other, and it's awful to witness, and it's awful to see that even though you love them well enough,

they *do* hate each other at times. Also, when you inter-
vene to stop the violence or the bickering, it gets worse.
Or they gang up on *you*. Aren't you used to your ac-
tions having more positive effects than these? Isn't it
absolutely stunning that your behavior can have results
totally opposite from those you intend?

Once you let go of the unrealistic expectation that
your children will always love each other, you can deal
with the fighting much more reasonably. You can say,
for example, that you know they hate each other now,
but they're not allowed to hurt each other. This puts
you in a more useful role—you keep them alive. It also
legitimizes the hate, and you've got to face the fact
that the hate, however fleeting, exists. No use telling
them that there's no such thing as hate. They know
baloney when they hear it. Haven't they heard you
cursing in traffic?

They hate you too, at times, and that's rough. But
it's the way it goes. The poor kids need help, and you've
got to give it to them. You've got to make the rules that
they love to protest (but love nonetheless), and it's just
part of the lumps you've got to endure that they can't
be made to *understand* you're doing the best you can
for them. There are limits to your being reasonable,
and, finally, it's reasonable to say "tough."

How come kids get sick when you try so hard to
protect them from germs? Don't try so hard, I say! It's
so much easier to be fatalistic about it. Should you take
your newborn to the international meeting of your profession when it happens to be in your town? Won't she
be exposed to wondrous bacteria and viruses? If your
pediatrician tells you that your baby is exposed to the

same crud at the supermarket, he is doing you a great service. Do you expend terrific effort preventing your baby from putting yucky things in his mouth only to have a cigar-chomping stranger breathe admiringly in his face at the drugstore? The baby has that nasty rash because he either inherited your allergies, has the chicken pox, needs to be bathed more often, is being bathed too often, needs more vitamin C, or is reacting to orange juice! You can't solve these problems, so you are hereby permitted to be relieved of the responsibility.

Injustice

The baby slept through the night two nights ago, but she didn't last night. She took a supplementary bottle of formula last week but refused it totally today. She nursed for five minutes this morning and slept four hours, but she just nursed for thirty minutes and is acting hungry again now. It's not logical. If you take it personally (and it's hard not to), it feels downright unjust.

Babies and children are great for turning you into liars. Your "shy" child of four years starts entertaining people on the bus while you ridiculously explain that she is not usually like this. Your six-year-old can't wait to go to the birthday party, and then he won't leave your side and cries painfully the whole time. You want to show off how your baby can speak a new word, but when it's time to perform, he acts like you're crazy.

The good thing about injustice is that it works both ways. You don't have to be fair. You send your child to bed at 7:30 not because she's tired, but because you need your evening alone. The double standard is great. Your child knows you're bigger than she is.

You know arithmetic, but your baby doesn't. When she falls asleep in the car during the last five minutes of the ride, won't she just naturally sleep the next fifty-five minutes in her crib? Doesn't work that way. She's equated that five minutes with a whole nap's worth, and you're out the respite you'd counted on. How many times have you put her to bed later at night, thinking she'll wake later in the morning? She wakes earlier still the next day, right?

You can so easily overplan and overdetermine. It's not worth it, because children change so fast that what is appropriate one minute is out of date the next. Not only do they grow incredibly fast, they are also notoriously ambivalent creatures who do not know their own minds (even when they are adamant).

You move to the suburbs because there is a fine school system, and your child will be able to walk to the local school. Terrific plan, but by the time he is in kindergarten, the town has closed the school because of underenrollment, or it's cut taxes so there are half the teachers there used to be. Or the school turns out to be great, but your son is jealous of all the other lucky kids who get to take the bus.

Regarding the "perfect" school, by the way—do you really have to sign up your baby for the progressive advanced reading preparation class before she's six months old? Some of the worst parental competition asserts itself in this area. All your friends are doing it, I know, but maybe you can consider relaxing, and not planning for it just yet. When it comes to schools, you'll have to take all kinds of things into account, not least of all your own child's reactions. For example, suppose you get her into the best school around, but for this year she has a teacher who is a dud. Or there are a few kids in the class who are disruptive or disturbed, and your child is afraid to go because of it. Or maybe everything is going fine at this superb school, and the thing your daughter likes best about it is the green and yellow tile that encircles the water fountain.

You don't get gratitude, either, so you shouldn't do the wonderful things you're going to do because you expect thanks. Kids always want more, and they reserve the right to feel cheated when they don't get the last thing they've asked for. It's impossible by definition to provide everything for that very reason. You go to the zoo, for example, and just this time you all get cotton candy, then peanuts, then soda, and on the way home you stop for an ice cream, and finally, when you're almost home, your kids see a toad hopping by the side of the road, and they want to stop and see it. You say no, and, boom, you're so mean they can't believe it. There's a rule built into children that commands them to wreck a perfect day no matter what, souring it for you right at the end. So stick to your guns, try not to make too much of it, forget about justice, and go about your business.

You do the best that you can. You love and you limit your child. And try not to plan *too* much.

Muddling
past the milestones

Intellectually you recognize that your baby's development is determined by his own very individual timetable. Well and good, except that it's impossible not to read the books that tell you when the typical baby is holding up his head, switching from bottle to cup, crawling, turning over, standing, walking, sleeping through the night, talking, teething, getting toilet-trained, and all that.

Parents eye one another's children for comparison, to check on how their kid is doing. Their child is smaller than yours and that makes you feel triumphant. But theirs is already using a spoon, and yours clamours incessantly to be fed by you. Shameful, no? No.

Milestones are probably vastly overrated. Is it really terrific that your baby has sprouted teeth? Looks cute and grown up, but now you have to work at feeling relaxed while you're nursing, and you have to teach your baby not to bite. Takes some doing.

Fabulous that she's finally started crawling, but now what do you do with the beautiful rubber plants that adorn your home? Baby proofing the place is a big pain in the neck. Paper clips, ant traps, staples, onion skins, kitty litter, electrical outlets, wood stove ashes, toilet paper, snow drippings—all offer a feast day for your little one. Wasn't it nice when she was sitting sedately, watching you cook?

Hooray, he's going on the potty by himself now! You are proud of him and he's proud of himself, too. But when you're in the car on the way to Connecticut, he needs to stop all the time to go to the bathroom. It's utterly beneath him to consider reverting to diapers for travel purposes. Or he's constantly interrupting you to have you undo his clothes so he can sit on the potty, and then you have to do him up again when he doesn't go.

There are drawbacks to reaching milestones, as the above examples indicate, but you get into more trouble when your child doesn't conform to the timetable of the "typical" kids (whoever they are). Is your child still sucking her thumb and carrying around that wretched teddy bear? It must be your doing that she still requires such "props"! Isn't she talking yet? Well, it's obvious that she doesn't *need* to talk because you provide for all of her needs. Why are people always pinning these things on *you*? Why can't they ever think of blaming the child? And, besides, who ever said it's so great when the kid starts to talk? It's hard to understand the words, and the child continues to be frustrated that she can't express everything. What's worse, you have to listen to her, and worse yet, she talks back. It's fine when speech is delayed, for whatever reason.

The best landmarks no one ever talks about. The ability to get one's own breakfast, for example, letting you sleep late on Saturday. Now that's worth pushing them about!

Ganging up on the baby

This chapter gives you the permission you need to "gang up on the baby." Once you have this permission, you will find that you'll be very good at it. You'll make up new strategies, new maneuvers, and new techniques that will give you a lot of pleasure.

If you've been reading carefully, you know that you've already been granted the permission to gang up on the baby. But this chapter makes it explicit, just in case you still have inhibitions, doubts, or lingering apprehensions. Dispel them!

The main reason you need to gang up on the baby is that you have to reassert the importance of your marriage. The two of you and your marriage are just plain vulnerable since the addition of your baby, and you need some fuel, some ammunition, to keep it clear who was here first.

You need each other as allies. Now imagine—you heard the baby crying at 2:00 AM, and you roused yourself, put on your bathrobe, nursed the baby with love in your heart, changed him, put him back, and are back in bed trying to fall asleep. You're drifting off, finally, when you hear him crying again. It's been a half-hour since you put him down—an hour-and-a-half, say, since you got up. The crying jolts you awake. Your husband stirs. The two of you wait to see if the baby is going to calm down.

The baby is twelve weeks old. He's not supposed to wake up at all during the night now, much less cry thirty minutes after the nursing. What's going on? What have you done wrong? Do you have enough milk? Is he going through a growth spurt? Is he teething already? Is his diaper full again? Didn't you burp him enough?

You and your husband groggily talk it over. The crying is getting louder, more insistent. The two of you just don't know what to do.

Well, I don't know, either. But one thing that helps is that you say *out loud* (this is the rule) the terrible, awful, unpublishable, unutterable things you think about the baby at this moment. "Maybe his arm is caught in the crib," you offer.

"Yeah, maybe his arm is caught and is twisting off," your husband adds.

Don't be shocked by what you or your husband say. It's outrageous, of course, but laugh and get some relief. It's fun to elaborate on these fantasies, too. Let them grow, multiply, get bigger and better. You're downright afraid, aren't you, that the baby is really sick, and that's why he's crying so much, but you also don't *care* right this minute, and you just wish he would leave you alone *now*. You're concerned about the baby, but there's a part of you that wants him to go away.

You're really mad at him at times. That's just all there is to it. It's good to recognize how angry you are at these times, and to share that anger with someone you love, and for both of you not to be too disapproving. It's all right to have these feelings. After all, you're *not* going to act on them. Venting them might just help you get through the moment and lets you feel better. Your fantasies can be so outlandish, so improbable and ridiculous that they make you laugh, and get you back to feeling like yourself quickly. Otherwise, you just might be fighting your frustration and irritation all the time.

Now do you get the idea? You can practice acknowledging your nasty thoughts on the blank pages in the back of this book. After you feel better, you can take care of your baby. You'll probably do a better job of it.

The new normal

While you are still terribly sleep-deprived, up once or twice or even three times a night, you can't see your way clear to life being "normal" or good again. You both are overwhelmed with the needs and the demands of the baby. The weeks go by, and it seems that it will always be like this. You will always be tired by the least things, and nothing will ever be the same again.

Some wonderful things are happening, too. You and your husband are growing to love this tiny infant. She is changing a lot from day to day. She becomes more responsive to you, and that is thrilling. One day the baby smiles; you're not sure that she did that, really, but as she continues to do it more and more frequently you know, and it is wonderful. The baby *smells* so good, too. The feedings are calming down; they are becoming special, nice times, and you feel so satisfied to see how the baby feels good after eating. You can almost see her grow before your eyes. When you think about it, it's already hard to imagine what life was like before you had the baby. It seems like she's always been around.

Eventually, eventually, the baby gives up the twice a night routine, and one night, maybe what seems to be eons later, she sleeps *through* the night. You can hardly believe it. It is like a gift from heaven. It feels so good. (Of course, you kept waking throughout the night, and if you are nursing, you feel incredibly swollen.) Nonetheless, it is truly a landmark. You probably won't feel nostalgic about those middle-of-the-night feedings.

Of course, she may not always sleep through the night from now on, just because she did it this one time. In any case, once the baby starts to do it more or less consistently, you are really going to begin to get some place. Only when that starts to happen, and you begin to get a cushion of uninterrupted sleep under your belt, do you make progress back to being normal again.

It's a new normal. Your lives have changed dramatically. You really can't imagine life without your child again. When you are away from your baby, you think about him. And there's a constant knowledge in you some place of the responsibility you have.

You don't have to feel terribly weighted down by this, though it's a big and enduring responsibility. Deep down in your bones, even when you've got the baby-sitter there for the afternoon, you know that you are not the free agent you once were. The morning you wake up with a miserable cold and a banging headache, you hear the baby crying, and your husband has already left for work, you *have* to get up to take care of her, no matter if you're sick or not. That's quite a realization. In the old days you could just call in sick. Not anymore.

At the same time, you may enjoy things more now. Before, you didn't know how wonderful it is to go out without the baby! When that babysitter comes and you and your husband go to the movies, the new-found freedom you feel is absolutely fabulous. And when you get home and the babysitter says your baby is cute, you can't wait to see him. When you're holding him again, it's just plain good. You couldn't have known these feelings before, and they're worth it.

Some nights the baby wakes up and cries. You wait and listen, wondering whether she'll go back to sleep. Eventually she does. It's quiet again. The silence is of a different quality than you'd ever known before: it's low and beautiful, smooth, cool and soothing. The baby who was just now crying teaches you this new appreciation of silence.

You and your husband are negotiating your new lives together. This process goes on all the time. It's good to remember that the two of you were here before the baby, and to put yourselves first every now and then. But everything is different now, and the routines that you used to have must give way to new patterns. As you begin to set up these new patterns—these new ways of being together, cooperating together—it gets easier.

Sometime in the first year (it's great if it happens early), your baby can give up the 10:00 PM feeding.

When that happens, you discover that you have your evenings back to yourselves! Pretty glorious. Eventually, too, you might lose some of the weight you gained. Eventually, slowly, your hips will return to where they used to be. Somewhere along the way you discover that you can have sex without the baby waking up and crying in the other room. Little by little, things get back to "normal."

You want to do some other things along with caring for the baby, of course. It will be a struggle, but it is possible. You feel it out; you wait till you're ready; you work it out with your husband; you learn about babysitters and day care; perhaps you push for flex-time and employee day care at work; and you see how to mesh everything. Little by little, you teach the baby and yourself that you are your own person as well as a mother. You feel out how much time you and your baby need to be together. (You both need time apart, as well.) And if you want to stay home with your baby full time, you still will be teaching him about your integrity as a separate person.

The baby is growing, and you are learning who he is. He's not quite what you expected. He's a new person, not reducible to someone else. There are so many charming things about your baby. He begins to reach for you. You know how to comfort him. As much as you're overwhelmed by the drudgery and boring pettiness of it all, you're increasingly aware of the miraculousness of having a baby. It's all in there together!

The three of you are now a family. Everything is now more complex and richer. Your baby has changed you from being a couple—working, loving, and planning—to being a family that has links to the past and to the future: to your parents and their parents, and to your child's children and grandchildren. Your brothers and sisters have become uncles and aunts to your child, just as you have (or will) become aunt and uncle to their children. Your baby has made you a family by linking you with all of them concretely. When everyone gets together, you see before your eyes how the children grow like weeds. This reminds you of your parents, aunts, uncles, and grandparents marveling at you so long ago. And on it goes.

And the three of you, the little group you now comprise—what a family you are! What traditions are you going to make up as you celebrate birthdays and holidays? What stories from your elementary school days will you pass on as legends to your baby? How juicy you'll make those stories about your mean brothers! Your child will listen enraptured, swallowing them whole, delighting then to tell his uncles on you! The songs you suddenly remember from the days your parents tucked you in you will sing to your child now. He can feel that continuity wrapped around him like a blanket.

The two of you look at your newborn, tiny in her large crib, and wonder. What ridiculously small toes! How could you have ever imagined her? It used to be just the two of you, and look what you've gone and done. Your love is even greater now; somehow it's stretched to encompass the baby, and the love the two of you have for each other has stretched, too—grown wider and deeper. Just look at the three of you! You two, the originals—once on a lark, planning, hoping, conspiring, not believing—now you're a family.

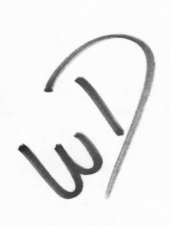